LOVED. LIVED. LOST.

IN SICKNESS AND IN HEALTH, TILL DEATH DO US PART

By Ghazala Jabeen

First published in 2018

ISBN: 978-1-5272-3247-1

Cover Photo by **Justin Van Marle**
Cover Artwork by **Mikyle Swindells**
Back cover photo by **Maddi Booth**

TEAMAUTHOR TA UK
Publishing with you

DEDICATION

This book is a tribute to my beloved husband Martin, who was my soulmate, my best friend, my mentor and now, my Guardian Angel.

This book is dedicated to our children, Mikyle, Charlie, Jennah and my step-daughter Jacky. It also wouldn't have been possible without the loving support from Steve, Adam, Stephanie, James, Jamie and my best friend Glenys.

These special people have been my strength and support and have kept me going during this difficult grieving process. I want to acknowledge how much I appreciate them all for their care, love and respect.

CONTENTS

FOREWORD

I feel humbled to be asked to write the foreword to this book. Though I never met Martin, I have known Ghazala for 6 years. We met through networking circles in North Wales and we clicked straight away. She has the most gorgeous smile, sense of humour and radiating personality - you can't help but feel something when you're in Gaz's presence.

As the 'Bollywood Queen', I asked her to help me celebrate at my 'special' birthday party in 2013. Little did we know at this happy occasion that it was the beginning of her years of struggle which she so poignantly portrays in the chapters of this book.

Gaz is a giver and a survivor. There's always something she's doing for somebody and even during the saddest time of her life, she focused on giving back. Raising funds. Marking Martin's memory. Being strong for her children.

In this book, Gaz lets us in on a side of her we don't often see - vulnerability. She writes with the same passion she gives to everything in her life, but through the following pages we see raw emotion as she shares the intimate details of losing the love of her life.

Family and friends are at the centre of Gaz's life and she is one loyal, strong and determined woman. Let's hope that this book will touch the hearts of the readers - to share with friends and family who are also dealing with a terminal cancer diagnosis. But may it also bring hope and courage to anyone struggling through personal tragedy.

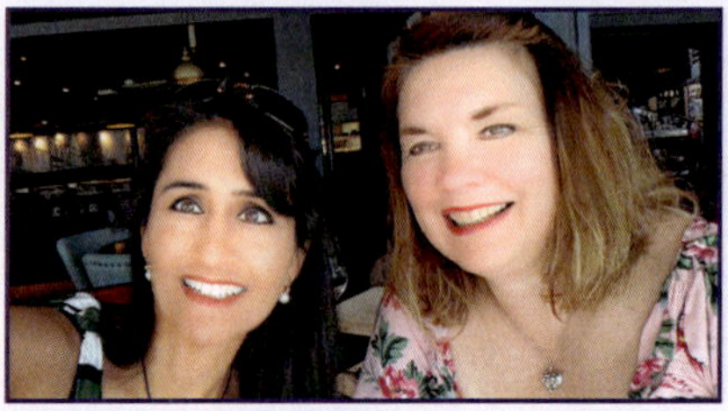

"Being deeply loved by someone gives you strength, while loving someone deeply gives you courage."
~ Lao Tzu

Susan Miller, Founder
Team Author UK

ACKNOWLEDGEMENT

Ghazala has been a huge supporter of Pancreatic Cancer UK for many years and we are so grateful for her unwavering motivation and passion.

In 4 years she raised over £11,000 through multiple charity events, organised awareness events by lighting up several landmarks in purple in North Wales and even launched a campaign.

It is individuals like Gaz and her wider support network of friends and family that can really help us to make a difference to those affected by pancreatic cancer in the future by enabling us to continue to provide support to those that need it, campaign for change and fund ground-breaking research.

We cannot thank Gaz enough for her support.

in support of

Pancreatic Cancer UK

www.pancreaticcancer.org.uk

INTRODUCTION

A love lost, a wish made and a mission accomplished!

It was 2014... a year to look forward to, marking some special milestones but everything changed!

Martin was my first love, he became my best friend, my soulmate and my everything. He and I had a wonderful marriage of 25 years. We had his mother Lily who lived with us, in fact she moved in to live with Martin a month before we were married. She was an amazing strong lady, who was looking forward to celebrating her 100th birthday. We had 3 children, Mikyle, Charlie and Jennah, 3 cats and eventually a little dog called Buddy that completed our family. We lived a happy life.

After a small fall, and years of ongoing tests and medical care...unfortunately, there was one test that changed our lives forever. We share our journey in how we dealt with our shock at the cancer diagnosis and how we learned to move on.

It was Martin's wish for me to raise as much awareness as possible about this cruel cancer. He set that seed of hope with a view to helping others and I continued to water that seed by raising the awareness with tremendous support from my family, friends and Pancreatic Cancer UK.

It is also about dealing with grief by opening my heart to share our journey through losing 3 loved ones in a year - two of which were to cancer. In the midst of all this, I was trying to stay focused on being strong and holding my emotions together. There were so many challenges in supporting my children, Jennah, Charlie and Mikyle (who's ages at that time were 16, 18, 20), yet all I wanted to do was cry on someone's shoulder. With an aching heart I was just hoping to find a way of dealing with it all but all I really wanted was for someone to say *it's not really happening*. It was like your ship is sinking and there is very little you can do to stop it. Then, you find yourself on a raft with your three children, fighting for survival and waiting to get to safety.

This book is written with the intention of helping others going through the dreadful time with a loved one who has been given that big bad word: 'cancer'. The chapters will cover some of the concerns we had to get our head around: the limited information and understanding of the seriousness of it. I will reveal the shock of hearing the news and the lack of care and support given to us. I'll share the symptoms and treatments and the unexpected changes to the condition, the family affairs, financial situation, the emotions and the whole process of the ups and downs of this awful part of our life.

It's my desire that the content of this book will bring some hope, help and strength to those going through similar situations. Regardless of the type of cancer, if you or your loved one is experiencing this dreadful disease, I want to help you find the resources, support and strength to work through this sensitive process.

Giving much love, light and respect to all who have been with me and my children throughout this time of our lives and supported my work with Martin's wish; thank you for recognising the importance of the message.

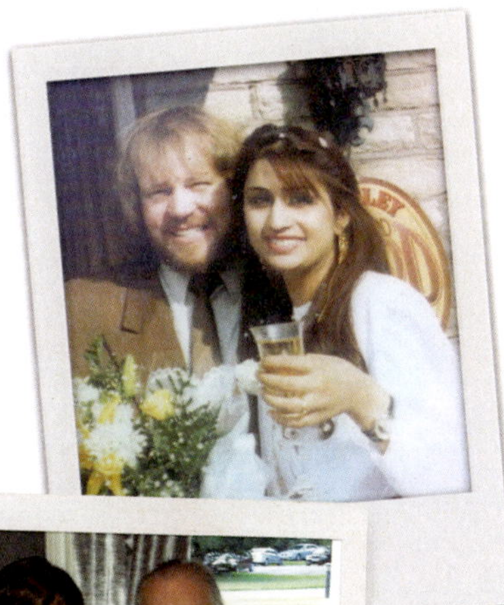

Be prepared to brace yourself as you join me on this journey with lots of emotions, anger and hope.

Ghazala Jabeen

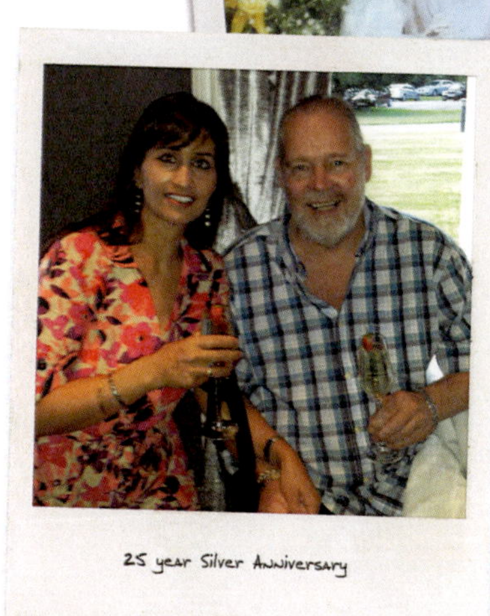

in support of

Pancreatic
Cancer
U
K

Chapter 1
WHAT IS PANCREATIC CANCER?

The pancreas is a large gland located behind the stomach. The pancreas is part of our digestive system and has two main roles.

1. It makes pancreatic juices which contain substances called enzymes. These enzymes help to break down food so the body can absorb it. The juices flow down the tube called the pancreatic dust, which runs the length of the pancreas and empties into the duodenum (the first part of the small intestines)
2. The pancreas also makes hormones, including insulin, which control sugar levels in the blood.

I hadn't even heard of Pancreatic Cancer or knew too much about the organ other than it dealt with releasing digestive enzymes and controlling glucose in our blood stream with the release of insulin.

The first mention of the possibility of the pancreas concerns was when Martin had dietary changes. There were certain foods either not settling in Martin's stomach or he would feel nauseated and started changing what he ate, which wasn't a balanced diet at all. This is what led us to go the doctors to find out why this was happening. Although we thought his stomach was damaged by taking too many prescribed drugs over a long period of time, in fact it wasn't the stomach issues as the main issue, but the pancreas.

Martin was seen by a Gastroenterologist to find out more about his stomach. Various tests, i.e. blood tests, CT scans and stool samples had to be ruled out but the pancreatic cancer wasn't confirmed until after a laparoscopy. This is keyhole surgery and a biopsy was carried out through the stomach to get to the pancreas. Unfortunately it wasn't very successful in getting into the pancreas but they were able to get some fluid and tissue from just outside it which was tested and confirmed that it was the pancreas affected by cancer. The specialist even said it was difficult to detect because Martin didn't have the usual symptoms that most people do that would have picked it up sooner.

Most people have some or all of the following symptoms:
Stomach pain or back pain, unexplained weight loss, indigestion (which Martin had), loss of appetite, feeling sick or being sick, bloating, burping or lots of wind, changes in bowel habits (ie, floaty stools) diarrhoea, jaundice, diabetes (diagnosed in the last year), pancreatitis (inflammation of the pancreas), gastritis (inflammation of the stomach lining) hepatitis (inflammation of the liver), gallstones, heartburn or chest-like pains, unpleasant taste in the mouth or even difficulty swallowing.

There are four stages of pancreatic cancer:
Stage 1: Earliest stage: The cancer is contained inside the pancreas but can generally be resectable (a possibility to remove or operate on it)

Stage 2: The cancer has started to grow in the duodenum (first part of the small intestines), bile duct or tissues around the pancreas, or in the lymph nodes near the pancreas.

Stage 3: The cancer has spread into the stomach, spleen, large bowel or into blood vessels near the pancreas and is usually locally advanced or unresectable (may not be possible to remove the cancer with surgery).

Stage 4: (The stage Martin's cancer was picked up) this is when the cancer has spread to other parts of the body such as lungs, liver, peritoneum (the lining of the stomach wall) this is called advanced or metastatic pancreatic cancer. It is not possible to remove the cancer cells once they have spread to other parts of the body but treatment is able to slow down the growth of the cancer.

Most people don't even know about these symptoms and often they are not picked up as a possible link to cancer and misdiagnosed as Martin's conditions were. He was being treated for depression, fibromyalgia, osteoarthritis (which he had as well, following his accident) chronic fatigue was put down as his weight problem and disability. In fact Martin's cancer was misdiagnosed about 15 times by our GPs and other specialists. Also, at our local hospitals there was not much in the way of literature or info leaflets in the waiting rooms. There were lots of take-away leaflets on other cancers and medical conditions, but nothing on pancreatic cancer. So I had to search on the internet to find out more about it.

This is where I came across Pancreatic Cancer UK and got information from them and have supported them ever since. They have helped me with everything from information leaflets, someone to actually talk to and all the things I needed when I ran fundraising events. I am very grateful for their support and understanding.

(Some of this information was taken with thanks from Pancreatic Cancer UK)

www.pancreaticcancer.org.uk
www.justgiving.com/gaz-jabeen

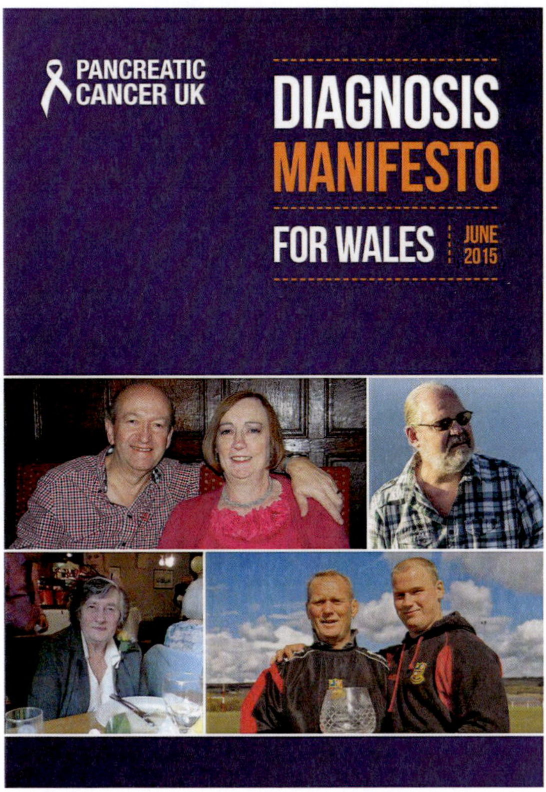

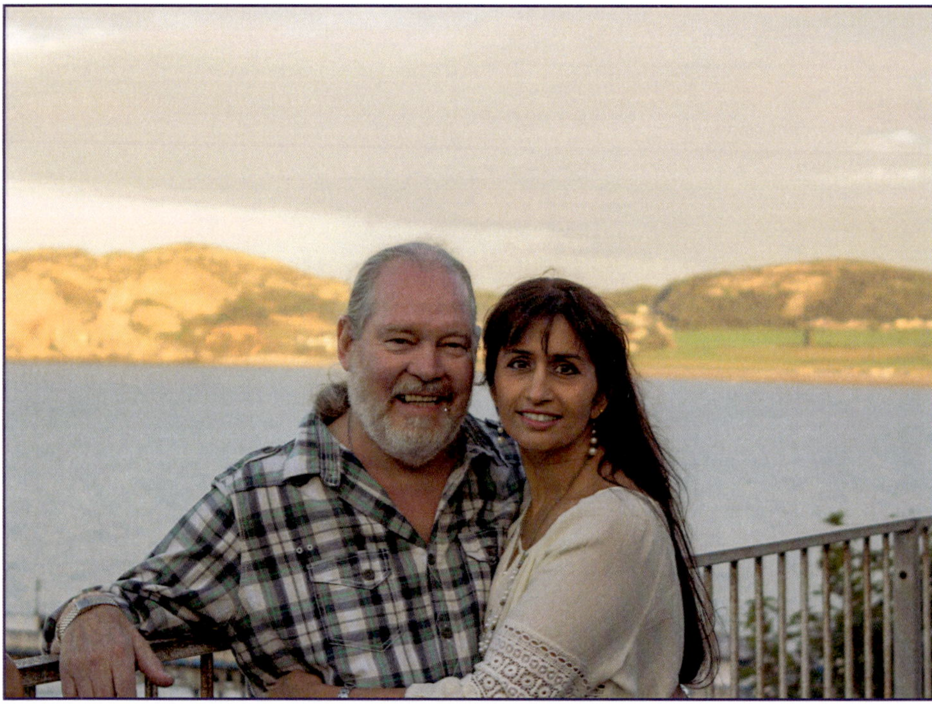

Chapter 2

A NEW YEAR, A NEW PLAN AND THE UNEXPECTED!

In 2014 we were preparing to celebrate our silver wedding anniversary...25 years of a happy marriage, especially with the challenges we went through to even tie the knot.

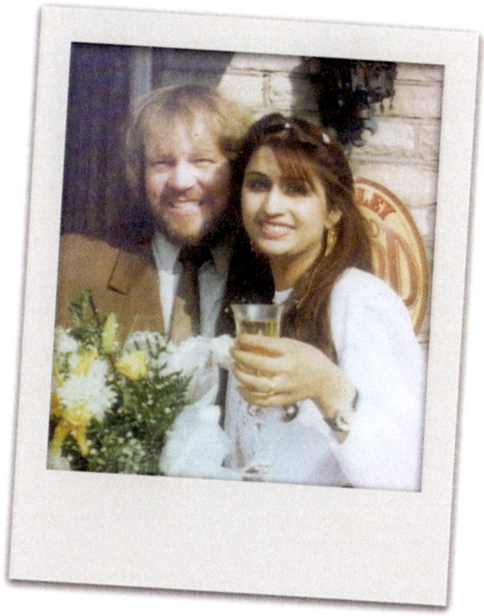

When I eloped with my first love at the young age of 20 to a man twice my age, my family were so angry, (in fact that is an understatement and is a story on its own, which I will share in a future book). They couldn't believe I had run away from home and said to people: she is young, naïve and silly and she will be back in six days. Well, six days went by, six weeks, six months, six years...and I didn't go back.

The year had started sad in some ways, as I was still grieving the loss of my father who passed away to cancer. Before my father died, he had eventually given his blessings and prayers and told Martin that he was a good, kind man. He said he was happy that he took care of me and we gave them three beautiful grandchildren. I was pleased that my dad and Martin had made amends before he passed away.

It was the 4th of August 2013, when my dad passed away. He had stomach cancer and though he had recovered successfully from the operation, the cancer had spread to his liver. I remember being with Dad in hospital when the specialist told him his liver cancer was at an advanced stage. My father's thoughts were very positive, and he said that this doctor was the best and would fix it all for him.

He didn't really understand what the true meaning of 'advanced stage' meant: inoperable and terminal. My sister and brother were with us and I remember feeling emotional just entering this private room to talk to the doctor. I noticed the box of tissues on the little table and thought a lot of tears have been shed in this room. We were just another family going through the process of this deadly cancer.

I remember sitting by my dad's hospital bedside right to the very end and even wiping his last little tear as he closed his eyes for the final time and took his last breath. It was so sad. I cried so loudly and hugged my mother to comfort her and got some comfort back from her too. It was the first time in my life I had witnessed death before my eyes and didn't know how to handle the situation other than to cry for my dad. It was all so final, tragic and simply heart-breaking. The whole family stayed strong together. We gave Dad a beautiful send-off with lots of prayers, love and respect for the incredible man he was in our lives and the wonderful teaching and upbringing he gave us.

Abdul Quayum
January 1940 – August 2013

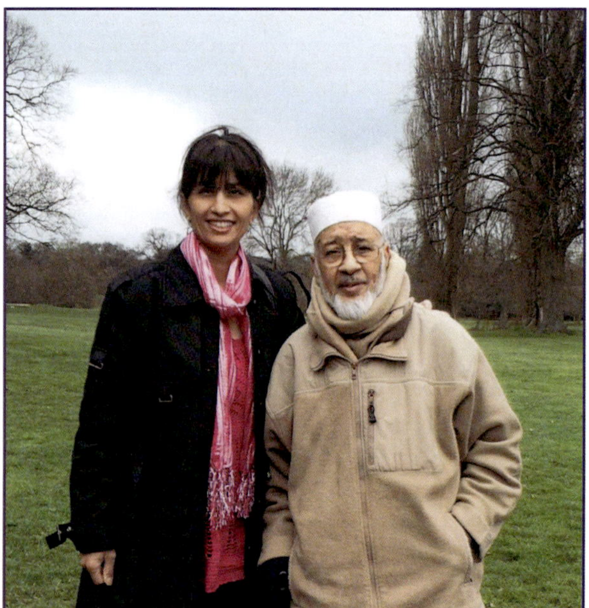

Chapter 3
CARING FOR MUM-IN-LAW

Dealing with losing my dad was one thing but also, all that travelling to Derby and back to Wales, I was so tired. I also had another big duty which was caring for my poorly mum-in-law Lil, who was 99-years-old and in her 100th year. Unfortunately, mum's health was deteriorating fast with old age getting the better of her. She was one of those who hated taking pills (she used to be a nurse and maybe knew different). She would say, 'Pain and discomfort comes but it will pass by too, just let it come and go.' One of her old-fashioned remedies to deal with headaches and pain was her Mackenzie's smelling salts. They used to nearly knock me out but she always had a little bottle by her side. She swore blind they did the trick. Bless her and her salts.

My mum-in-law was a big lady and trying to physically move her around or help her up was very difficult. We were advised by doctors to put her in a home, but Mum was having none of it, so Martin and I decided to care for her as much as we could at home by ourselves. Mum had very funny ways and was very particular about her food. She used to say that she preferred my baked potatoes and main meals to Martin's because he never put enough salt to flavour it. She would moan that his meals would be late and she liked things on time, especially meal times. She never seemed to understand that Martin was running around sorting the children's meals too. This was something that both Martin and I were not very good at: being on time, because we were running our business and needed to have flexibility with things we did. The funny thing is, she would barely finish her current meal and ask when the next one was being served. She was a much regimented lady and very smart in her appearance.

I remember I used to always ask her opinion on things especially when I was getting dressed to go out. One day she was left shocked and in laughter bearing in mind, English being my second language, I used get sayings a little bit wrong. Martin would often say, 'Go on Wifey, put on a nice sari and let's go out for dinner'. On this occasion Martin had bought me a few new saris and I chose one and got all 'togged up'. I went into her room and said, 'Well Mum, what do you think? Am I dressed up like a dog's end or what?' She nearly fell off the chair laughing. I didn't know what I had said that was so funny but she couldn't stop laughing. She said, 'You mean 'a dog's dinner' – Not a 'dog's end'!' I saw the funny side of it and there was I thinking I was getting better with my English sayings.

However, back to Mum's condition; sadly she was getting worse with her mobility and she ended up getting cellulitis. We had to call the doctor to the house as she couldn't walk much, or even get downstairs. He prescribed her some antibiotics and asked to have a quiet word with us.

He suggested that she should go into a care home as it seemed too much for Martin and I to start lifting her physically. She would need proper medical equipment and aids to help her within a proper environment of care.

This became a tough decision for us because we knew that a nursing home was the last place Mum wanted to be in. We decided that we could care for her at home with some assistance from carers and nurses to help deal with her daily needs. So, the plans were put in place to do exactly that.

Martin and I were very tired, and Martin hadn't fully recovered from his MRSA infection (which I explain more in Chapter 4). He was still on a lot of medication. I was working flat out to provide for our family. It was tough going but we persevered as much as we could. Mum was certainly very challenging, especially when she wouldn't take her medication and I literally had to sit by her side for ages until she plucked up the courage to do so. Unfortunately, her condition was getting worse and deteriorated fast, and she was fully aware of this too.

One day she said, 'I never knew the day would come that I cannot do things for myself and end up in this sad way relying on others to keep me going.' She felt very depressed because she didn't like the way she was living. I'm sure she felt like time was catching up with her and I could see such sadness on her face. It was etched with fear and helplessness. I really tried to keep her uplifted with my daft conversations and would get the odd smile at times, but it was not easy.

Martin was brilliant in caring for his mother. From the day he decided to have his mother move in to the house until the latter part of her life, he went beyond the duty of a son to give his mum the very best he could in her senior years. She didn't want for anything and was very grateful for this. One day she said, 'Martin, one of the best things you've done in your life son, is marrying Ghazala. She has been good to me and always a breath of fresh air.' It touched my heart to hear this because Mum didn't always say what she thought.

I recall once when she was sat in her wheelchair feeling low, she fancied a nice cup of tea. She would have it black with one sweetener, so I happily went to make that for her. When I brought it up to her and was about to go, she said, 'Don't go just yet, stay here with me a bit longer.'

I said, 'I would Mum, but I've got lots of ironing to do.' She told me to bring my ironing board into her room so she could have some company. It made me realise she was getting really scared of being alone. So, I stayed with her a bit longer. I then mentioned it to Martin and the children to spend more time with her and so we took turns, taking shifts to keep her company. I also told the children to tell her what they'd been doing all day, telling stories or any chit chat that would make her feel better. Jennah would take Buddy our dog up to see Nannie as she loved him so much too. This became the pattern of care to keep her going. Mum always used to say that Mikyle, Charlie and Jennah were her reasons to live. She adored the children so much and always treated them to things, from their favourite foods to clothes or things they needed to help them with their studies. They loved their time with Nannie too.

Then one day Mum's leg gave way and she could no longer support her own weight. This meant she now needed to go into hospital where proper hoisting equipment needed to be used to care for her. We had to call 999 and the ambulance arrived in less than 10 minutes. The paramedics went upstairs to see how they could help get Mum downstairs and into the ambulance. This was a tough process, not because of getting her downstairs but because of her fight not to leave. Her words still haunt me as they helped her to the ambulance. She said, 'I don't want to go to the hospital because I will never come back out alive.' Bless her, she was so worried, but knew it had to be done as we just couldn't manage to hold her weight and physically manhandle her at home any more.

When she was in hospital, we notified the necessary families and they all paid her a visit. We were busy arranging 24-hour care for her to go into a nursing home, as there was a shortage of beds in the hospitals. She was in Glan Clwyd and Colwyn Bay hospitals in North Wales. Unfortunately, the care at both was not very good. There were situations where they left the band on her arm after taking her blood pressure. She had to tell us that there was a band on her arm that was causing pain. We found the staff in both hospitals to be unhelpful and when Mum tried talking to them and asking something, they would not always respond to her. She would tell us that they ignored her on so many occasions. I remember one evening when we went to see her, we noticed that the oxygen bottle was empty and there was Mum relying on it. The staff were not even aware of this. It was shocking some of the poor quality of care from these hospitals, in our opinion.

Just before getting her into a nursing home, I went to see her one evening with a little something to eat, as she liked me bringing a few things that she liked such as a baked potato with cheese and onion. I noticed a bunch of flowers on the bedside cabinet. I said, 'Hey Mum, I see you've had visitors?' She pointed at the note on the flowers, as she couldn't speak properly with her oxygen mask on and looked very tired. I read the note and it said:

Dear Ghazala,
I want to thank you for all you have done to look after me in all these years, especially the latter part of my life.
Mum x

She had me in tears for this kind gesture in her poorly state. She had asked our children, Charlie and Jennah to pick up the flowers from a local shop on their way back from school and asked Jennah to write the note. She was keen to show her appreciation for me, even in her poorly state. God bless her.

When I finally found a beautiful nursing home for her, I was so pleased that it was new and had the best equipment and care facilities in place. She fussed about everything from the room being too small, she couldn't see much out of the window etc. We eventually settled her in and she was on 24-hour oxygen but getting very confused.

A few days after being in the nursing home, I got a call from them to say Mum had an accident and could I get to the nursing home as soon as possible. We made our way as soon as we could. They explained that she had slipped from the hands of the carers and fallen in the bathroom. So once again she was totally confined to bed. Sadly a couple of days later she was not being very responsive. I was working away in Chester when I got a call from the nursing home to say Mum had gone worse and it was important to be with her now. My heart sank when I heard this. I told Martin to get to the hospital right away and I drove to be there from Chester. Our children Jennah and Charlie went straight to her after school, but Mikyle was at university and couldn't be there until later. When I walked into Mum's room Martin was sat holding her hand and the kids were in the room looking very sad. Martin then said he couldn't face seeing his mum die in front of him and left the room. I went over to Mum and talked to her to reassure her that I was there and to breathe properly from the mask. She gripped my hand but seconds later she took her last breath and died right in front of my eyes. The kids were in shock. I pressed the buzzer and the nurse came and confirmed that Mum has passed away. I held the kids and we all cried like mad. I phoned Martin to let him know; he knew himself it was imminent, but he wanted to remember his last time with his mum as asleep. He kept that thought of his last words to her as he held her hand and could remember her being alive the last time he was with her.

Lily Swindells died peacefully on 27th May 2014, nine months after my dad passed away. It was a tough time seeing two people close to my heart die in front of me.

We gave Mum a wonderful send off and our house was full of flowers; in fact, it looked like a florist's. It was not easy receiving flowers being delivered to the house because some were being delivered for my birthday which was on the 30th. Some were delivered with happy messages and others with condolences. It was a strange and sensitive time to receive these beautiful flowers.

Mum was cremated, and our three children paid an excellent tribute in the eulogy for their dear grandmother with such wonderful words of what she meant to them. They did her proud. Martin and I asked the Vicar to say special words from us for this amazing lady.

In this moment I pay tribute to a wonderful mother-in-law who was like a real mother to me. I had become so fond of her over the 25 years I had known her and she had taught me so well. We had wonderful times, from learning to make a good English gravy to what I wore. She was a strong and a very proud lady admired by so many who all called her 'MUM'. God rest her soul.

Lily Swindells
October 1914 – May 2014

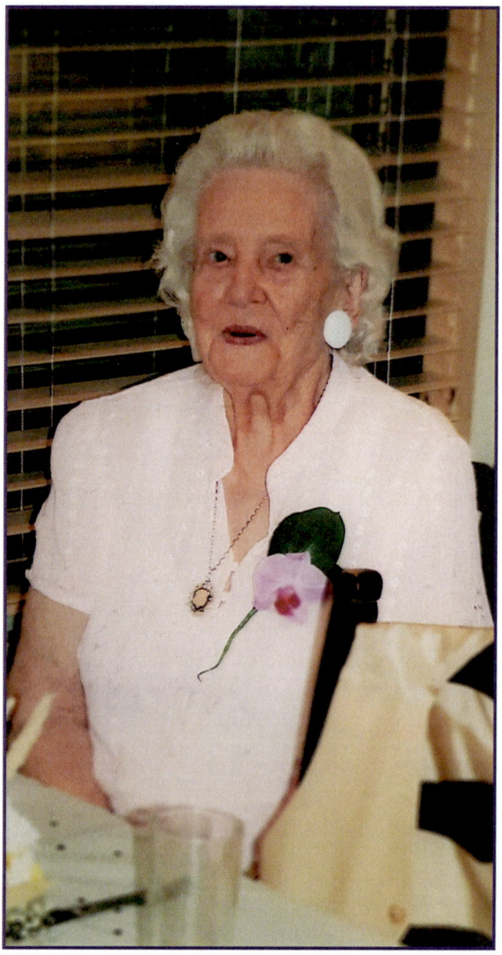

Chapter 4

MARTIN'S FALL
(GOING BACK TO OCTOBER 2010)

After Mum's passing, Martin and I sat and had a rethink of our plans and made the necessary adjustments in our home. We removed the stairlift and re-did the walk-in shower room and removed all the disability equipment around the house.

Much of our time had been spent caring for Mum respectfully to the end. It inevitably brought a lot of stress and tension through lack of sleep and worry, so perhaps it was time to take some time out for us. A little TLC wouldn't go amiss, especially as it was coming towards our 25th wedding anniversary. We thought it was like starting our marriage over again with a clean sheet of paper. The kids were nearly all grown up too and it was our time to enjoy some special time together. We had put 'us' on the back burner in order to care for our family.

One of our plans was to travel around the UK (Martin was not into flying) and we loved Cornwall. I suggested we spend some long weekends away for us to energise, rest and rejuvenate.

I started to look at some cottages in Cornwall and Devon with a sense of a new chapter in our life. When I would mention some dates to Martin about going away, he would say, 'Wifey I am tired and don't feel well; let's organise it next weekend.' This went on for a bit and I didn't actually get round to booking anything. Martin was spending a lot of time sleeping and looking lethargic and kept apologising for not being well enough to travel. I would say, 'I am not surprised Martin, after all the stress we've gone through.' Martin had lots of health issues and his body was really tired out. We had mental, physical and financial stress as our income had drastically dropped whilst in caring roles and in particular after Martin's fall.

On a cold, crisp October evening Martin and I decided to go for a little drink at our local pub, the Pen-y-Bryn, which we did quite often, but on this occasion, it was a little different. I had made one of Martin's favourite curries and we decided to have it when we got back. When we finished our drink, the staff (Gareth, Adam and Georgina) at the pub said they were hungry and were going to order some late-night food. I happened to mention my curry and suggested that they were more than welcome to pop over to ours for a midnight meal, instead of ordering pizzas. This was very tempting to them as they all knew of the famous 'Gaz Curry' and Martin encouraged them to come to ours too.

Our house was like the hub of the community and everyone was always made welcome anytime. After all, when I make a curry it is never a small pan...it was always enough to feed an army.

They were delighted and came back to ours for a little midnight feast. We laughed and enjoyed our time eating curry and talking about fun times. When they were leaving, Martin went to see them off safely. Upon his return to the house, he slipped by the front door (drink had nothing to do with this as Martin was driving). He stopped himself from falling to the floor and pulled himself back up. When he came in, he said he pulled something behind his knee and decided it would be ok in the morning.

The following morning, Martin couldn't move his leg properly and said his leg had seized up and he couldn't even stand on it. I called the doctor to the house. She came and realised how bad Martin's mobility was and suggested Martin go into hospital and arranged for an emergency admission by ambulance. He was admitted to the hospital and was diagnosed as having a torn ligament. He was told to rest it and then would probably need some physiotherapy. Martin was back and forth with this problem but unfortunately, he fell again and was taken back to Bodelwyddan Hospital, only this time things were not administered properly.

Meanwhile, I was working to keep our business going and to earn enough to keep the bills paid. After work I phoned to see how Martin was doing so I could go and see him or bring him home. However, they couldn't trace where Martin was. I said, 'How can you lose a patient?' I told them that he was admitted by emergency ambulance but they couldn't find where he was transferred and asked me to check admissions. When I did, they said there was no one with that name admitted on any ward. They said he may have been taken home. I said, 'How?' They said they didn't have that information either. I said, 'He would have only been taken home by me but I have been at work all day.' I was so worried by this time that I drove up to the hospital to find out what on earth had happened to my husband. I had to leave our son Mikyle to sort the kids' dinner while I was gone. Mikyle said, 'I can do pizza Mum, since it's the easiest to do.' So I told him to be careful and I went off to hospital A & E reception. They couldn't understand where Martin was transferred but they did have him on record to say he came in as an emergency case by ambulance. I decided to head over to admissions reception and to my shock as I walked down the corridor, I saw Martin on a stretcher with a thin blanket and he was laying in an awkward position. I couldn't believe that he was just dumped in a corridor with no one knowing where he was. Martin said he had been there ages and had no way of calling anyone for help. He was desperate to go to the toilet and his neck was hurting from sleeping in an awkward position. I was so angry and asked for some help. Martin was then transferred to a ward. He was in a bad way and began telling me that he had had a knee procedure with an injection and to aspirate the knee and a steroid injection to reduce the pain.

One of the things that Martin told me was that he found it odd when the surgeon did the procedure, he opened the packaging and put on the sterile gloves and then said to Martin, 'I better close the curtains,' which he did with the gloves on and carried on. Martin knew that this was not correct practice because of the dust falling off the curtain and other potential germs that could transfer to these sterile gloves which were in place for the needle procedure straight after.

Unfortunately, Martin contracted the MRSA bug and his CRP levels were extremely high. He needed to be put on intravenous antibiotic drip.

Meanwhile, I was still working my job and running my Bollywood classes and I would end up visiting Martin after my classes in-between feeding the kids and Mum, settling them down then driving up to the hospital. Then one evening I went to see Martin and he seemed very spaced-out and not making much sense. He looked so poorly and weak and was hallucinating saying that there were cats on the ceiling. By now I was wondering how many drugs they had given him and why were they not keeping an eye on him, checking he was eating his foods properly. I asked the hospital staff and all they said was he didn't want to eat and they couldn't force the patients. This was concerning to see how badly his health was deteriorating with more drugs in his system than food.

By now Martin was in the hospital for nearly 3 weeks and all the family were getting deeply concerned on why he wasn't getting better. Martin's mum said, 'I haven't seen my son for nearly 3 weeks and I want to go to hospital to see him myself.' Bearing in mind Mum hadn't been out of the house for a very long time. I told her I would get her a wheelchair sorted and take her.

I took the children first and asked Martin if he needed anything specific bringing. He said, 'The tea in the hospital is awful.' (Well he used stronger words than that). I knew he liked a McDonald's tea, so I went to get him one.

I then arranged for the family to visit and made arrangements to bring Mum in a wheelchair too. It was Martin's daughter Jacky, his son-in-law Steve, Mum, our children Mikyle, Charlie, Jennah and our close family friend Glenys. We thought he would feel at home and better seeing us all. When we got to the ward, he was fast asleep. We sat and waited for a bit and then I started to talk to him and he opened his eyes and looked phased out. I told him that Mum was here too. He was not responding very well to us at all. He kept nodding off and coming round. He called me to him and said could I ask everyone to leave as he couldn't cope or concentrate, it was too much for him. So, we all left his bedside and sat in the canteen and talked about how much he had gone downhill. Mum was so worried and said she had not seen her son look so unwell and felt very sad, as did all of us.

A couple of days later, the kids and I went to visit him, and he agreed to us bringing him a 'Big Mac' and another tea, which we did. I remember when he started to eat his food, he was 'wolfing' it down like crazy. After all, he hadn't been eating properly for weeks. Then Jennah said, 'Dad can I have a bite of your burger?' Martin nearly bit her head off saying, 'No, it's mine!' He was so protective of his burger. We realised how starved he was for some food with some taste. So I took some McDonald's meals for him and he started to get better with more energy about him. Eventually he got well enough that the hospital said he could go home.

I had asked on several occasions to speak to the specialist to see what had really been going on with Martin but I was not given much support or information. The nurses would say the specialist would explain, yet every time I got there at the agreed time, they would say he was doing the other wards so I never got a full explanation as requested. I felt his care in the hospital was so poor and truly felt he could have died if I hadn't taken him some extra food to help him get some energy back to fight it. Finally, Martin came home and was looked after with extra loving care and was fighting strong again. He was however, not fully able to walk and so we had to do follow up appointments to see what was next on the agenda to get him walking again.

When we went back for a follow-up appointment, I was ready to ask the specialist all the important questions I needed answers for, but that specialist was no longer on the case. We were told Martin would be seen by another orthopaedic specialist who happened to be one of our neighbours. We explained to him how unhappy we were with all that had been going on and asked him to take us under his care and help get things better, which he did.

He explained that Martin had picked up an infection and it required further antibiotics to bring the CRP levels down and that the medication would be a lot stronger, involving 2 different types of antibiotics at the same time to fight the infection. He also explained the risks involved ie, damage to muscle, tissue, bones, brain etc... It was that, or Martin would never walk again and the infection could get a hold and make things worse. So, with limited choice we had to agree to get the necessary treatment to fight it. We had our worries about the strength of these drugs and the length of time it was going to take to see how it would affect Martin in the long term too. We felt we had no choice but to brave the decision and face the consequences.

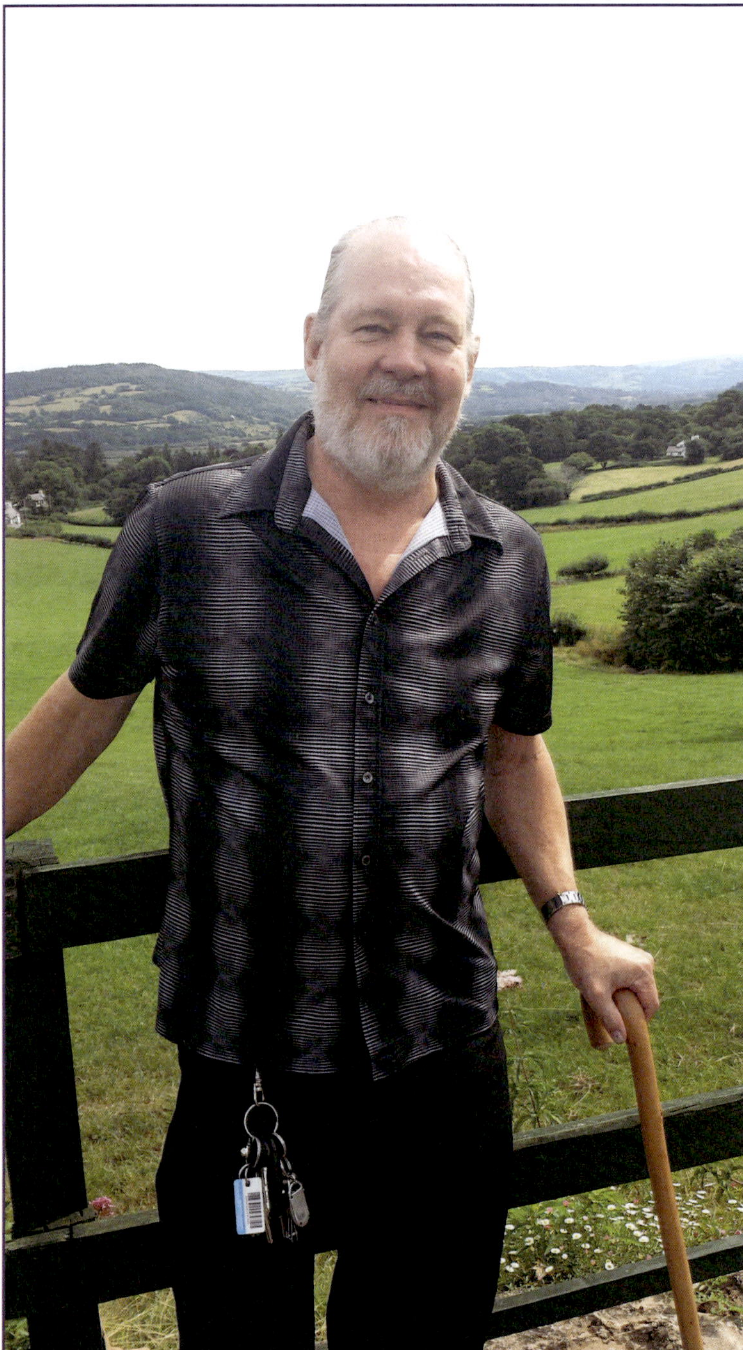

Chapter 5

THE DIET CHANGE

Our plan of spending some time out to celebrate our 25 years of life together wasn't going as well as planned. Our journey had taken a different direction altogether.

Martin just kept feeling poorly all the time; he kept saying that he couldn't eat certain foods and I tried to adjust my recipes to fit his needs. I was shocked though when he said, 'Wifey, you know I married you for your lovely curries, well I can't eat them anymore.' I jokingly said, 'I thought you married me for my lovely hair. If that is the only reason you married me, does that mean you want a divorce?' He laughed and said, 'No Wifey, we have come this far and we shall continue the journey together to the end.'

Martin's eating habits kept changing, especially when he started having Shredded Wheat for breakfast, Crunchy Nut Flakes for lunch and Weetabix for supper. He would say that they settled with his tummy better than spicy or greasy foods.

Then one day Martin came downstairs with a big smile on his face and said,
'Guess what?'
I said, 'What?'
'You'll be glad to know my weight is going down very nicely!' This had been a major problem to shift because of Martin's lack of mobility.
I said, 'That's great, but it's not a well-balanced diet is it? You can't live on cereals every day.'

Martin had been to the doctor so many times about his chronic fatigue and general run-down situation. He was sweating a lot and not able to focus on doing things. They diagnosed him with anxiety and depression and put him on more drugs, including treatment for what they said were symptoms of fibromyalgia. I was once again concerned about the amount of drugs he was taking and the effects they would be having on his body.

When he kept saying his tummy just wouldn't settle, I replied by saying, 'I am not surprised with the amount of drugs you have been prescribed.' I said he should go to the doctor and ask to be referred to a specialist.

So, when we got to the hospital, I spoke to the nurse about our concerns and she said she would mention it to the specialist and made a note on the file. Whilst we sat in the waiting room, we saw our Gastroenterologist walk by and we smiled and tried to say hi. He looked at us and totally ignored us in a very arrogant way, which left us wondering what we had done wrong. To make things worse, the nurse came to us and said there was a delay in the appointment times, because they were having some technical issues with the probe that was used. 'Please bear with us and we will call you when we are ready.'

This left us even more nervous than before. In fact, we just wanted to go home at that point, like it wasn't meant to be, but we persevered. When Martin eventually got called and headed towards the area for the procedure, I went with him to talk to the specialist about the needle worry. The senior nurse said that I didn't need to go as she would be going through that herself. She told me to go have a coffee or something and come back in about 45 minutes. So, I did but felt ignored a bit. When I got back, Martin had been gone a long time and still wasn't out. One and a half hours went by and when I checked with the receptionist, she said she would find out and let me know what was happening. Then one of the special nurses came to me and said that the procedure had taken a bit longer and Martin had come round too quick so they had to sedate him again to finish the procedure. Now he was sleeping off the medication but should be out soon. Martin eventually came out and there was a nurse with him. She gave a brief update to say that there wasn't anything to worry too much about, there was some inflammation but at least it wasn't the big bad 'C'. We were reassured but Martin seemed to still be very light-headed from the medication and we slowly walked out of the hospital. He said whilst we were walking slowly down the corridors, that it was an awful experience because when he came round he was choking on a pipe down his throat. Obviously the medication to sedate him wasn't the right amount for the procedure to be given again. Surely, they should have gauged that better knowing what was involved.

The following day we got a phone call from the specialist's secretary saying that they would be getting in touch with us following the test with which day Martin could go in to discuss it. She said they would phone us and double-checked which number would be the best to call on. She also said that it would be in the next few days. It felt like there was something going on for it to warrant a telephone call and that our appointment was going to be in a matter of days.

A few days later, I had a Bollywood event booked on Anglesey and I said to Martin, 'Fancy coming along for the drive and we can take Buddy with us?' I thought it would be nice for him to go for a run out especially as Anglesey is beautiful and it would be good to have a nice day out together. He agreed that it was a great idea.

I used to moan at Martin for doing so much sleeping or watching repeat programmes. He would say, 'Leave me alone, I think I am dying.'
My reply was, 'Well, we are all dying from the minute we are born.' I would complain about the amount of paperwork that needed doing and he would say, 'Stop nagging me Wifey, I will do it in a bit.' I remember once saying, 'Martin, you sound like a grumpy old man and you need to pull yourself together.'

At times I would feel I couldn't cope with all this stress of running around like a headless chicken feeling tired and drained. Sorting Mum, kids, the business, the home, the admin etc...

One day my neighbour Iain said he saw me struggling to bring the shopping in looking very tired and realising that nobody was there to help me. He even said he thought Martin was lazy letting his little wife run around doing this and that and he was not helping out. I just smiled at Iain and told him he wasn't feeling well. We continued to wait for the results to see why he was so low. The situation was also getting noticed by our children wondering why Mum and Dad didn't seem happy with each other at the time. I was thinking, *I don't want to leave this man I love but I am finding him difficult to cope with*. I was so tired and this was the last thing I needed to think about.

I then phoned my best friend Glenys to say I needed to meet up and have a coffee and a chat. As always, she was there for me and made her way over. We met half way at McDonald's and got our coffee and sat in my car. I opened my heart out to her and described what I was dealing with. She could see my frustration and the sadness in my face and she said she didn't know what to say or what to offer as a solution. She only told me afterwards that she prayed that we wouldn't split up, because she knew we had a special relationship.

We took a little moment and shared a chocolate muffin (saving some calories). She did however, say something that I felt was touching. She looked me in the eyes and said, 'Gaz I got my ears to listen to your troubles, shoulders for you to shed your tears on and my company to comfort you.' For me, this was just the little pick-me-up that I needed at this very trying time just to share and halve my worries with a friend whom I could totally trust and open up to anytime. I cried, I shared and I talked until I couldn't anymore. I felt lighter just off-loading my concerns and came away feeling a little lighter and feeling I could handle the situation a bit better.

The trip to Anglesey eventually came up and off we went, Martin, Buddy and me. It was a lovely run out. Whilst I went to do my Bollywood dancing, Martin took Buddy for a little walk. I came back and then we went for a coffee and enjoyed our little chat. I wanted to capture our nice time together by taking a picture, which I did and as I looked back at the picture, I said to Martin, 'The picture is nice, shame about the background.'
He said, 'Why, what's in the background that you've captured?'
I said, 'A Funeral Director's and a cross.' (It was like the writing was on the wall).

We finished our coffee and drove up to Camaes Bay and parked by the dock. As we watched the boats and people leisurely going about their business, we got a phone call; it was the specialist's secretary saying that they had an appointment date and wanted us to go to the hospital in 2 days. The MDT meeting would have finalised the necessary report by then. As soon as I heard the term 'MDT meeting' it sent a shiver down my spine, because the last time I heard that term was when my dad was diagnosed with cancer. I knew it was the term for a specialist team coming together to discuss the best plan for the patient, usually in the event of serious ill health such as cancer. This worried me a lot. The phone was on loudspeaker and I didn't want to ask any questions about my concerns at that time. I didn't want to worry Martin on something that might not be what I was thinking. As we were driving back, Martin said, 'What's that all about then, Wifey?', to which I replied, 'Not really sure Martin but we will know about it in 2 days' time, after they collate all the info properly.'

Although deep down, I had a sinking feeling but kept a brave face as we made our way home from Anglesey.

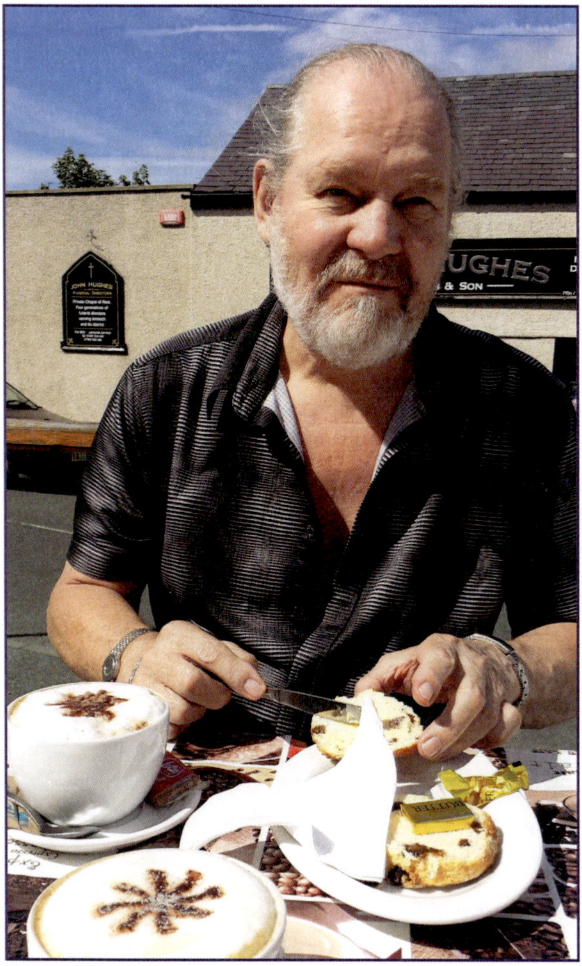

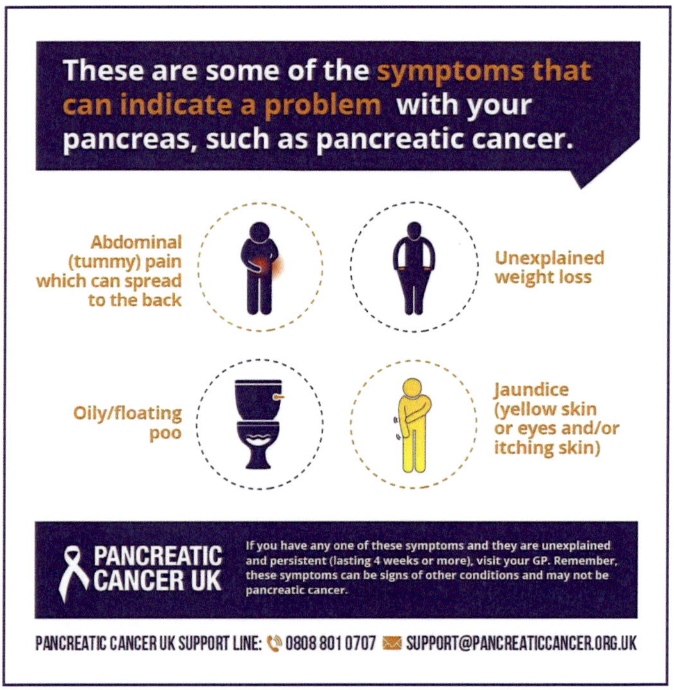

These are some of the symptoms that can indicate a problem with your pancreas, such as pancreatic cancer.
Abdominal (tummy) pain which can spread to the back
Unexplained weight loss
Oily/floating poo
Jaundice (yellow skin or eyes and/or itching skin)
PANCREATIC CANCER UK
If you have any one of these symptoms and they are unexplained and persistent (lasting 4 weeks or more), visit your GP. Remember, these symptoms can be signs of other conditions and may not be pancreatic cancer.
PANCREATIC CANCER UK SUPPORT LINE: 0808 801 0707 SUPPORT@PANCREATICCANCER.ORG.UK

Chapter 6
THE DIAGNOSIS

On 23rd July 2014, we had an appointment with the specialist. We were both apprehensive about what we would be told but keen to know what was really going on so we could deal with what was required to improve Martin's health.

We were invited in the room by the nurse and sat with the Gastroenterologist who looked at us both. Then he looked at his notes, he flicked his file notes back and forth a bit while Martin and I sat and looked at each other. Then the specialist said, 'Well, Mr Swindells, we have all the results back now and spoken to other specialists too, and unfortunately it's not good news.'

I remember my heart stopped beating for a minute. I was not sure I was ready to hear what news he was about to deliver to us. Martin seemed in better composure than me. We looked at each other as though silently agreeing between us that we were ready to face this together.

The specialist continued and said, 'We couldn't get a biopsy of the actual pancreas, as it was difficult going through the stomach to get at it. However, we managed to get to the fluid around the pancreas and it has been tested. It seems that you have a rare form of Pancreatic Cancer, as you have not shown the typical symptoms that would have been picked up, such as jaundice, pain in the abdomen etc...'

I remember being a bit numb after hearing the word 'cancer'. I quickly reached towards Martin and held his hand. He was still so composed and said to the consultant, 'What does that actually mean, I mean is it curable?'

The specialist turned round and said, 'Unfortunately it is what we call advanced stage.' We were still not clear what that meant. We needed to know how advanced and what was to be done to help treat it.

The specialist said: 'It's terminal.' After hearing the word 'terminal', the tears just rolled down my face and I started to sob thinking, *this cannot be happening*. Martin squeezed my hand and said, 'I told you that I was dying.'

I said, 'Oh, Martin stop it, don't say that!' I couldn't cope or comprehend with what we had just been told. At that time, I was hearing but couldn't listen to what else was being said. I turned to the specialist and with tears running down my face, feeling heartbroken and with a quivery voice I asked, 'What kind of treatment can help and what do we need to do?' I wanted a thousand questions answering, but unlike me, Martin just wanted basic bare facts, as he was always a very matter of fact kind of guy.

He looked at my sad face and looked at the specialist's straight face and said to him, 'I want to know what kind of time I have got? I need to know so I can make the necessary provisions for my wife and my children and I need to know.'

The specialist said he would be passing the file onto the Oncologist who would be dealing with it. 'He will be the one looking after your case now and I doubt I will be seeing you again unless they call for me and my assistance. You will be seen on the 25th July.' (two days' time) He added, 'I am sorry that I am the bearer of this sad news and I wish you the best.' He shook Martin's hand and said goodbye and escorted us out of his room.

This process left us shocked and saddened deeply, in fact it was one of the lowest points in our life. To make it even worse was that not only are you told that you have the big bad 'C' but then be told it's not curable and not have any nurse or someone to support us after this devastating news was awful. Not even a cup of tea or sit down or a discussion straight after other than goodbye and wait for your next appointment.

Martin and I held hands and with heavy hearts walked down numerous corridors making our way out of the hospital. Martin didn't say much to me and I didn't know what to say to Martin either, in fact we couldn't believe what we had just been told or what to do next. Talk about life just going all 'blank' on us. One thing I knew was that everything was about to change and nothing was ever going to be the same again. The unknown territory was very scary indeed.

On our way out there was a Macmillan Cancer Support booth with information leaflets and books, so I headed towards it to find out if there was one on Pancreatic Cancer. I couldn't find one, but did find some that I felt would give us some advice. They were on chronic fatigue, financial situation, and other general things, but nothing specific to what we had to deal with. I picked them up and grabbed Martin's hand and we continued out of the hospital. My legs felt all shaky and my stomach was churning with stress but all I wanted to do was stay strong for Martin. We got to our car and I gave Martin a big hug and said, 'I am so sorry darling for this awful news they have given you, but we will fight this together and stay strong through it all.' He had sadness on his face but as always, he just smiled and said, ' Wifey, thank you for being in my life and thank you for being you.' We got in the car and I just cried and couldn't drive off straight away. Martin cried too and then we just hugged each other to comfort our hurt and sadness.

After ten minutes, I pulled myself together and drove off. Our home was about 20 minutes from the hospital. As we joined the A55 expressway, I recall Martin looking at me as I tried to brave the journey home. Unfortunately, I wasn't being brave, because I pulled up at the services and parked. Martin said, 'What's up?'

I said, 'I can't cope.' I was shaking and trying to deal with the shock. I said, 'Let's go in the café and get a strong cuppa before driving home.' Martin agreed. We got a tea for Martin and an Americano for me and I took a few sips as we sat looking at each other. 'What are we going to do?' Then I couldn't help my tears flowing, feeling that this wonderful man that has been my best friend, my soulmate, my partner, my everything is not going to be around anymore. I couldn't sit in a public place and be in a mess. I said, 'Come on Martin, let's go and sit in the car.' Instead of Martin being in a mess like me and me trying to console him, it was him trying to console me. It was an awful situation. I took lots of tissues from the café because I didn't have many in my car and I certainly was going through them.

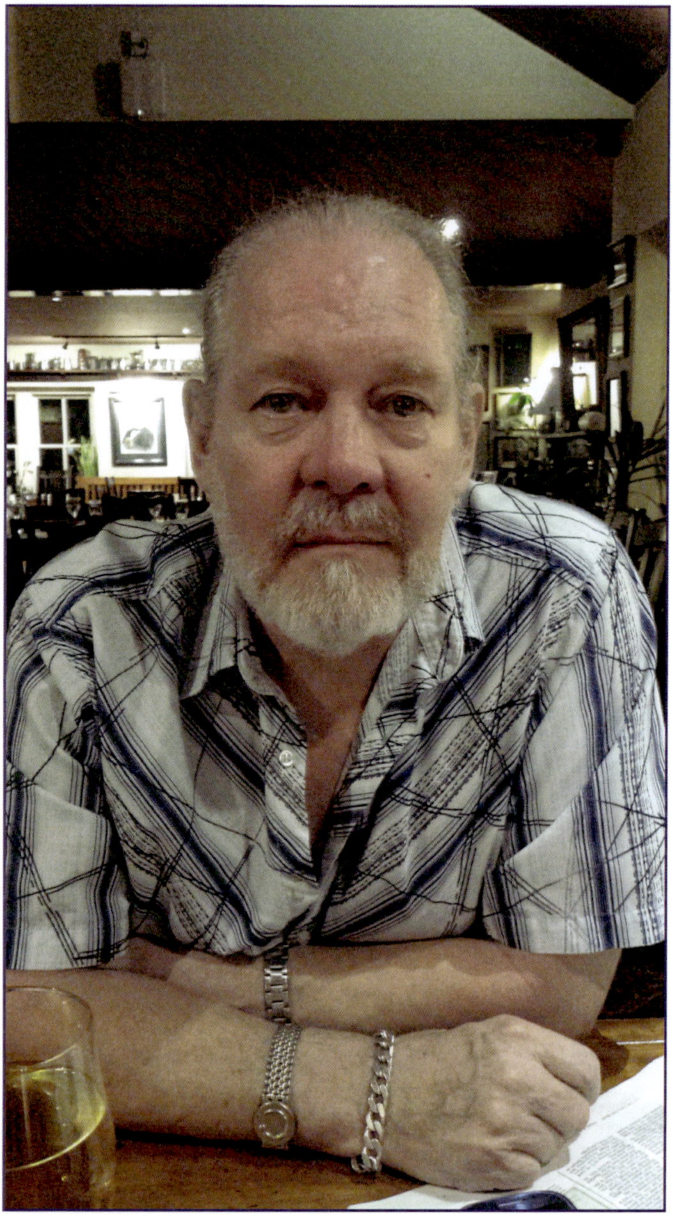

Chapter 7
MARTIN'S THOUGHTS

When we got in the car, Martin said, 'We need to phone Jacky.' (Martin's daughter) who asked us to let her know how we got on with our appointment. He also said we needed to get our three children (Mikyle, Charlie and Jennah) together to tell them too. So I messaged them to tell them to be at home for 7pm. Then he broke down in tears.

I said, 'What's made you cry?'
He said, 'This is the worst thing to deal with.'
I said, 'The cancer?'

'No, telling the kids. How on earth do I tell them that their dad is dying? I cannot bear to see their faces with this news and how will they cope, especially when anything needed fixing or they needed answers to things I would be there.' He knew they always went to their dad for so many things and relied on him for help as they grew up. Their dad was the man that would always find a solution and to know that he wasn't going to be around would be a terrible blow for them. I realised that this had really hit Martin hard now. The reality had sunk in.

We sorted our emotional state and finally dialled Jacky's number. She answered in a concerned way and said, 'Well, what have they said?' When we told her the details, she got very upset but once again, like her dad, she kept a strong composure. She was so sorry that this was the findings and knew it was going to be difficult telling the kids about it. She suggested coming up after work and being with us to help deal with it. After all they were her younger brothers and sister and they looked up to Jacky with lots of respect. We agreed that if she didn't mind, then that would be helpful.

I then phoned all three of our kids and repeated to them to be at home for 7pm and that their dad and I wanted to talk about something very important. I also said they mustn't be late or be rushed to get back out. I remember Charlie asking, 'What is it all about? Give us a clue at least? Are we in trouble?'

I said, 'Son, if I answer one question you will ask me another and it's not fair on the other two, so please don't ask any more questions, just be at home at 7pm and we will go through it properly with all of you.'

A 6.30 pm, Martin's eldest daughter turned up and gave her dad a big hug and then we sat and waited for Mikyle, Charlie and Jennah to arrive. Eventually, one by one they got home, saying they'd been thinking all sorts as to why Mum and Dad wanted them home. When they saw that Jacky was there on her own, they realised this was a different kind of meeting.

They kept saying, 'Have we done something wrong?' They also feared that perhaps Mum and Dad were going to split up or something or maybe they were going to surprise them by taking them to Disneyland. I asked them all to sit down. Jennah sat next to Jacky, I sat next to Martin, Charlie sat next to me and Mikyle sat on the chair next to Charlie. Then there was an uncomfortable silence.

This I knew was going to be such a sensitive situation and really didn't know how it was going to be said or heard. My heart was racing but also on guard to be ready to protect the kids from their hurt and to stay strong for Martin too.

Martin took a deep breath and said, 'So kids, you know when we call you all together you are usually in trouble, right? But on this occasion, you are not!'

Charlie said, 'Phew, thank God for that. I was worried sick as to what we had done wrong.' Then Martin paused and I knew how hard it was for Martin to come out with this devastating news. I just squeezed his hand as if to say *I am here with you, you can do it*. Jacky also left her chair and walked over to her dad and held his other hand. The kids looked terrified at was happening.

Martin said, 'It's not you lot in trouble, this time your dad is in trouble.' The kids looked at each other as if to say, *what are you on about, Dad?*

Martin continued slowly. 'You know I have not been well for quite some time now and I have been going for many different tests. Well, today they confirmed what is wrong with me. Unfortunately, I have been diagnosed with pancreatic cancer and sadly it is advanced stage which they confirmed means it's terminal and there is no cure.'

The kids' faces froze, and I remember Martin said he looked across the room to Jennah's face and said, 'I can't forget Jennah's face and her beautiful brown eyes, over-flowing pools of water as she tried to understand the seriousness of the news that her dad was going to die.' She then leapt off her chair and threw her arms at her dad and sobbed her heart out. Charlie and Mikyle did the same. We used to love our family group hugs but this one was not the same. This was one was very different.

It was certainly one of the most sensitive and most hurting time in our lives. Our happy home was broken and the one person we loved with all our hearts was going to be leaving us forever. How would we ever cope and move on without our Martin? These were the thoughts and feelings going through us. We were beside ourselves with emotion, frustration and anger at the situation. Our world had just crashed right before us. Our big man with the big heart would be leaving us. We were left broken, angry and terrified with the enormity of what we had to face on the next part of this journey. Our worst nightmare.

The evening stayed heavy on our hearts and we just tried to comfort each other the best we could through this difficult time.

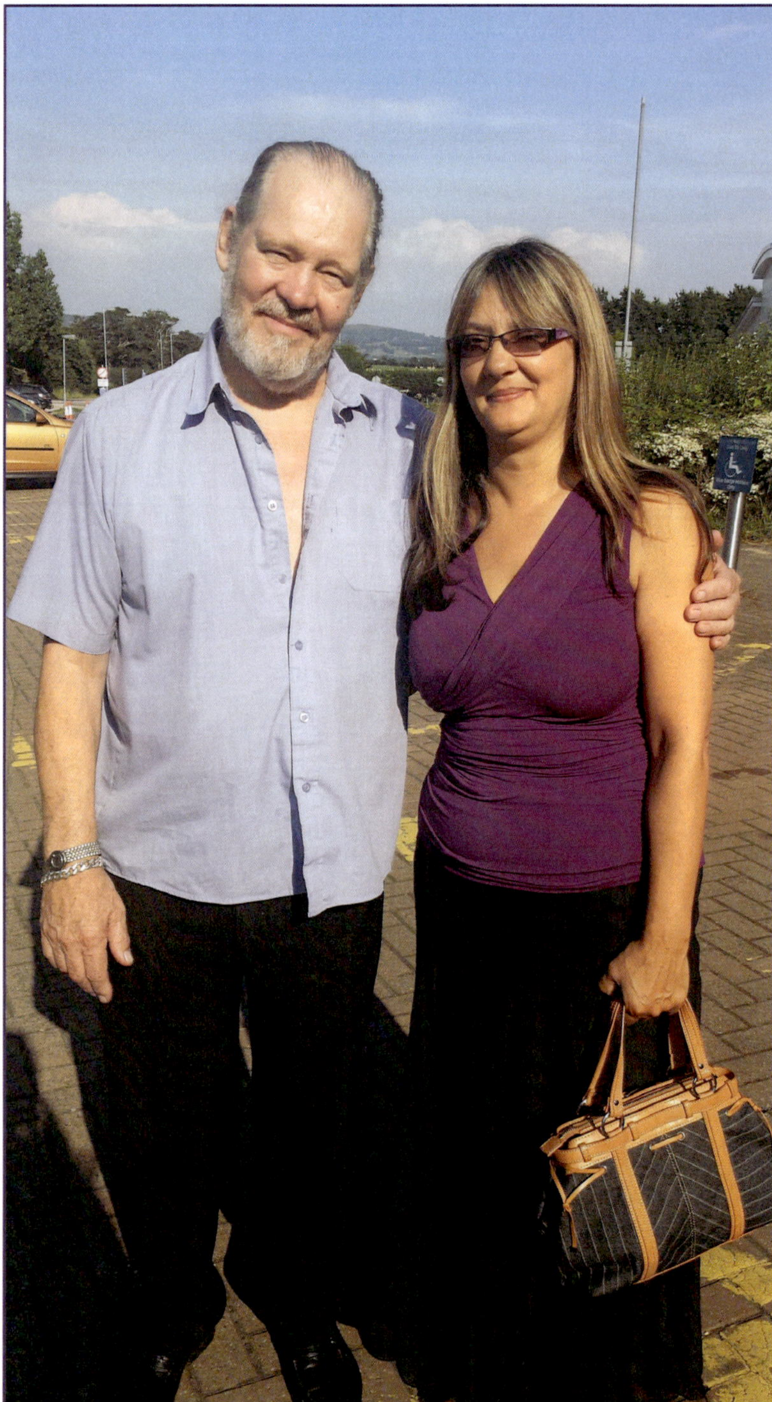

Chapter 8
THE ONCOLOGIST

It was appointment day with the Consultant Oncologist, where we'd be told exactly what the findings of the tests were and what treatment and process we would have to go through. Once again, Martin's daughter Jacky stepped into support us and was there with us at the appointment so she could take notes in case we missed anything.

The Oncologist confirmed that the tests showed that Martin had advanced stage of Adenocarcinoma – in short, a terminally ill condition with pancreatic cancer. Martin asked the Consultant how long he had based on the stage he was at, even with the necessary treatment. He wanted to gauge some timing on his situation. The consultant explained, 'Based on everything we are treating and the current drugs and treatment plan for your condition, we are looking at approximately 11 months.' Once again, the truth hit us hard because we thought Martin might have had a few years still.

Jacky's face was *OMG!!! Is this really happening?* She made as many notes as she possibly could and kept her best posture through the appointment. Jacky has always shown great strength even when she has felt upset and sad inside. She always has a look of 'we can deal with this', just like her dad, being very matter-of-fact about things.

At the end of the meeting, the Consultant started talking about dates to see how early we could get Martin on chemotherapy treatment and start to put the process in place. He also mentioned that there were signs of swollen lymph nodes and signs of concern on some spots on the lungs too.

During this investigative process and plans for Martin's treatment, I was still running our business, looking after the home and running my Bollywood fitness classes. It was so very difficult to keep a happy face in class. I was trying to keep the students uplifted and motivated, yet deep in my heart I was hurting so much as my world was crumbling. The song 'Tears of a Clown' was going through my mind. I was marching on like a brave soldier for everyone and all I wanted to do was to shut the door on everything and cry. I just wanted everything to mend or turnaround or they tell me that they made a mistake with it all. I was also suffering from a foot injury, with a fallen arch, plantar fasciitis and a heal spur. I was under a specialist to have my foot treated. As if that wasn't enough, I was travelling back and forth to my mum's which was about a 3-hour journey to deal with her hospital appointments and the paperwork at her home since Dad passed away. It was like one challenge to another and it just didn't seem to be easing at all. I didn't have many choices, so putting aside my own aches and worries, I kept going to deal with what needed doing, praying for things to get better, hoping for some kind of miracle to happen or someone somewhere would listen and step in to help me.

On Friday the 1st August, a week after seeing the Oncologist, we had another follow-up appointment to see him. He asked how Martin was feeling and Martin mentioned about the numbness in his fingers and that he kept dropping things. His grip was not strong and he explained about getting very frustrated whenever he would drop things and they would break. He was angry at his condition and not really knowing how best to handle it. The Oncologist thought that there may be something pressing on the spinal column and we needed to rule out any possible tumour growth there too. He was very efficient on acting on this, especially on a Friday afternoon. He arranged an emergency MRI scan. He even escorted us out to the MRI department and told us to wait there when we were done and he would come back to see us. I sat and waited in the waiting room observing the unhealthy-looking water filter machine where all the staff were filling their bottles of water, thinking their mouths have been on their bottles and they are all sticking the bottle top in that filter machine, adding their germs to it. It just didn't seem right or hygienic. Anyway, under normal circumstances I would have written a complaint or questioned it but right now I was dealing with my husband's terminally ill condition whilst he was undergoing an emergency scan.

When the scan was done, Martin came out looking very dizzy after lying in the machine for a bit. Soon after, the Oncologist turned up and went to grab the report and asked us to go the private room at the side of the scanner room. He sat and went through it and then looked at Martin and said, 'Well the good news is that the spine looks well and there is nothing indicating any tumours or other problems that relate to the cancer.'

Martin said, 'Well, that's something. It's the only test that has come back ok. How re-assuring.' He also said to the Oncologist that his problem with his grip was an issue and the best way he could describe it was it was like when people have a stroke and the brain is doing one thing and the body is not responding to it the same. The Oncologist advised us to book an appointment with our GP and ask for an urgent referral for a brain scan to see if there was anything there that we needed to look at. We agreed and left the hospital on a mission to tackle the next test.

I booked another appointment with the GP and explained all the information giving a full update on what we had been through. The GP said he had had some letters sent from the hospital and was aware of the circumstances. He was sorry at what we were going through and referred Martin for an urgent appointment to have a brain scan as requested by the Oncologist.

The brain scan was done and we had to wait to be notified on what to do next. Our normal Oncologist was away on leave so we saw another specialist. It was a lady Oncologist who sat with us to explain the results. She said, 'Martin, we have found a couple of tumours on the brain and one is big and the other one small. It does also indicate it is secondary cancer on the brain. However, we need to look at your plan again regarding the chemo and the possibility of radiotherapy.' She said that Martin's main Oncologist would be back the following week and it would be best to see what his advice was and follow on from that. She was reluctant to discuss much more with us at the time.

We left the hospital a little unsure on how much this would change the treatment plan, and it was another bad blow to be told that the cancer had spread to the brain. Another area of uncertainty on how we would move forward.

When we went to see Martin's Oncologist to discuss the brain tumour scan, he explained a few scary truths to us. Martin said he wanted the honest truth of the real picture for us to work with. So, the Consultant said, 'Sadly one of the tumours is quite large and this alters the time frame a lot.'

Martin and I looked at each other and our thinking was, *how much more bad news can we take?* The Oncologist said the 11 months' time we looked at before had now decreased to about 3 months, because of the brain tumour. He said we couldn't do the chemotherapy at this time, we would need to address the brain situation urgently and that involved radiotherapy. 'I am going to refer you to the Radiologist and they will explain what comes next.' He also explained that the reason this was more urgent is that it would be the brain cancer that would kill him before the pancreatic cancer. He also explained that it would also depend on how strong Martin was after the treatment before we could look at chemotherapy.

Each time we went, Martin had a regular blood test, weight check and other checks to see how he was managing and his general wellbeing. The doctor explained that radiotherapy could also kill the good cells in the process of destroying the bad ones. Martin very bravely said, 'Well let's do what needs doing and hope for the best.'

Chapter 9
THE BUCKET LIST

After our hospital visit, we went straight to the bank so Martin could pass the power of attorney to me and let them know that he couldn't write very well. A new signature was needed on all the documents. Everything was being changed around and time kept reminding us that it was like an hourglass and we had so much to sort out before the sand ran out.

Martin's other big concern was worrying about the work that needed to be done to the big beautiful red Bentley that I had bought him for his birthday. He wanted to get the necessary work done to it in order to sell it. He started doing some work on it himself. I kept telling him he shouldn't be worrying about these things and that we could get someone else to do it and he would reply, 'Wifey that would cost more money and I know what needs doing. Remember, time is running out and I can't leave you in this mess. I need to do what I need to do, after all I am dying so I might as well get on with things and know I have done my best. If we can sell the Bentley, it will give you some money to work with until you get your feet back on the ground again once I am gone.'

This was the horrible truth to face, but it was what we did. I would stand by Martin whilst he fixed the car. I would stand there with a spanner in my hand or some kind of tool to help him and watch over him to make sure he was ok and to help him up when he would lay under the car to look at what else it needed doing to get it ready to sell. I remember both of our sons Charlie and Mikyle spent time with their dad whilst he tinkered about the car and couldn't help but think, our boys are going to miss their dad so much when it comes to fixing their cars and spending time in the garage. Just doing what boys with cars do, tinkering with tools in engines, oil and grease and the fun they always had. It was a picture embedded in my head and captured for life. A sad but lovely picture of our sons loving their time with their dad as he loved his time helping his children learn from him.

When we got our appointment to go and see the Radiologist, our daughter Jennah (who was at home because of school holidays) said she would like to come along to the hospital to support her dad, so we agreed she could come too. When Martin was called and we both stood up to go in, Jennah said, 'Can I come and see your brain scan too, Dad?' So we checked with the specialist and he said no problem. I asked Jennah if she was sure about it as it might upset her, and she said, she was sure and would learn from it too. Her future was to be a vet and she was interested in understanding what scans were all about and how a specialist reads it. Jennah has always been very matter-of-fact with things, another child who was just like her dad.

When we sat to watch the screen with Martin's brain scan, we looked deeply at it and tried to make sense of it but obviously it wasn't that clear for us to know what we were looking for or what to read and where to look at the areas of concern. Then the specialist pointed out the dark patches; one was a big one and another small one. The Radiologist also explained about the brain membrane and how it works and why chemo would not help the brain cancer and vice-versa. There was so much to learn and get our head around all this information.

Now time was not on our side and everything was in full flow from appointments and treatments. We didn't even get time to digest things or ask questions because we had to do what was necessary to try and treat the cancer quickly and stay strong and positive throughout the process.

Steam Rally Car Show - Chelmsford

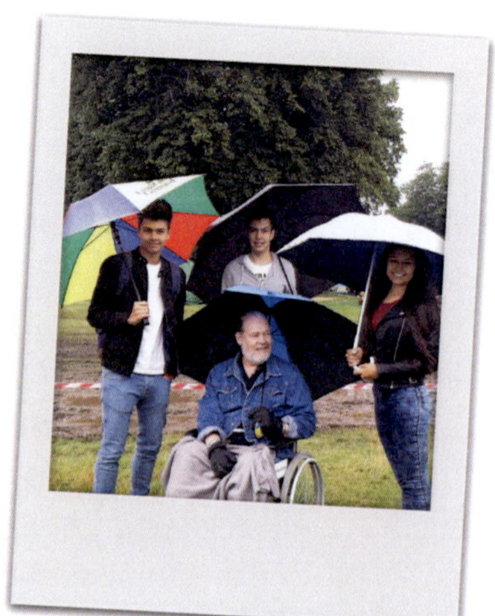

We realised that with the limited time frame we had in our life, we needed to make the most of the things that Martin wanted to do: His 'bucket list'. I asked Martin what kind of things he wanted to do so we could plan to do it for him. He said one thing was to go to Chelmsford to the steam rally car show. He said that in our married life it's something we would have wanted to do every year and because I wasn't that into it, he never got to see many of them. So, I planned for us to all go there. I also knew that Martin was not well enough to walk around the place and asked the district nurses that were looking after him at home where and how I could get a wheelchair for the weekend. They asked me to contact The British Red Cross, so I contacted them and explained the situation and they organised for me to pick one up from Abergele. I gave a donation to them for their support.

The day we were set to travel to the show happened to fall exactly on our 25th anniversary (10th August). It was raining very heavy and we had a struggle parking our car on the field. Then the next part was to see if we could push Martin and the wheelchair through the muddy field. Oh my, what a job that was. Martin's 16 stone weight, mud and lots of rain was certainly an obstacle course. The children and I took it in turns to push the wheelchair and managed to get around the car show. Martin loved sharing his knowledge about the cars with the children. He seemed so happy to be there regardless of the rain. Actually, the rain didn't dampen our spirits – it added a lot of fun for us and we didn't moan about it at all. I captured some pictures of Martin and the kids scoffing burgers and laughing and enjoyed watching everyone having a great time. It was a special moment captured with lots of love for each other.

Double Tree Hilton - Chester

Another event which was very special was to actually spend time out for our 25th Wedding Anniversary. It was fortunate because we had won a gift voucher from a RSPCA fundraising event. It was for an overnight stay at the Double Tree Hilton hotel in Chester with dinner at the Marco Pierre restaurant and full use of the leisure facilities. Martin, Jennah and I used to be volunteers at the RSPCA for many years and always supported their events to help fundraise and help out at the centre as much as we could. This voucher was one I kept and thought it would be a nice treat for us, but with all the things that were going on with Mum and then Martin, we never got to use it before. When I rang the hotel and spoke to the Manager, I explained about the length of time that had gone by to make sure the voucher was still valid and that I wanted to book a special time away for our anniversary. I explained Martin's condition and the reason for the delay. He was a wonderful Manager and he honoured the voucher and said not to worry about anything and that all would be sorted and that they looked forward to seeing us.

It was booked and we were looking forward to some relaxing time for us on our own. When we turned up at the hotel and went to check in, the Manager came out specifically to welcome us and said they'd laid on a couple nice surprises for us to make our Silver Anniversary very special including a special duo spa treatment. We were delighted and checked in and headed off to our room. When we got to our room, there was another lovely surprise waiting which was a personalised cake with 'Happy 25th Anniversary' written on it. We felt very special with that lovely touch.

We then went down to use the leisure facilities and the Spa treatment centre. When we were filling in the details and paperwork which asked lots about medical conditions, the therapist said she was not comfortable doing a massage for Martin because of his condition with the cancer and didn't want to disrupt the lymph nodes or anything that could make his condition worse.

Martin said, 'Look, I only have so many weeks to live so there isn't any more you can do to make my terminally ill condition any worse.' He said he would sign the paperwork to that effect and with that reassurance, she decided to do a gentle relaxing massage for Martin. We had a duo room and looked into each other's eyes as we lay there, side by side. When the therapists finished they placed our hands together and left us to have a moment to ourselves and to come through when we were ready. It was so tranquil and all I could think of was wishing if only we could have many more years together with more wonderful experiences like this. We then went into the relaxation room to listen to sounds of the waves. We enjoyed sitting quietly listening to the sounds of the ocean. From there we went back to our room to get dressed to go for dinner.

When we arrived at the Marco Pierre restaurant, there were two glasses of champagne ready for us and the waitress escorted us to one of the nicest tables for two in the restaurant right by the window overlooking the fountain in the garden. It was so romantic and just perfect. The waitress came over to our table with an envelope on a silver tray. I wondered what that was all about and Martin said, 'Come on Wifey, open it. You know you like opening envelopes.' It was an anniversary card from the chef and the staff to say *Congratulations* and to ask for anything that we needed to make our experience a wonderful one. We were very touched by this lovely gesture. We had a delicious meal but when it came to our dessert, Martin and I couldn't make up our mind which to have, the choices were all enticing! We asked the waitress what she recommended and she agreed they were all lovely and tasty. She asked which ones ticked our box, and then said, 'Give me a minute,' and went off. The next thing we knew, she was back with a big plate with all of the desserts in mini sizes for us both to share! She said if we couldn't finish them all right now, she would wrap them up for us to take to our room. I thought wow, what excellent service. They couldn't have done more for us if they tried. It was certainly a special time for us.

Classic Car Show - Tatton Park

The following day we met up with our children at another car show. This time Martin walked a bit more but also had his walker fame with him and rested every now and then. The day was enjoyed by us all, seeing how happy Martin was. It was sad too, knowing this might be the last time he did this. We took so many pictures. Martin knew so much about the cars and specifications on the different models that the kids were impressed and learnt a lot from him. We asked the kids to take a picture of us two in front of a classic Rolls Royce to say we made it 25 years. We had had a picture in front of a classic Rolls Royce when we first got married. It was a wonderful, memorable day out.

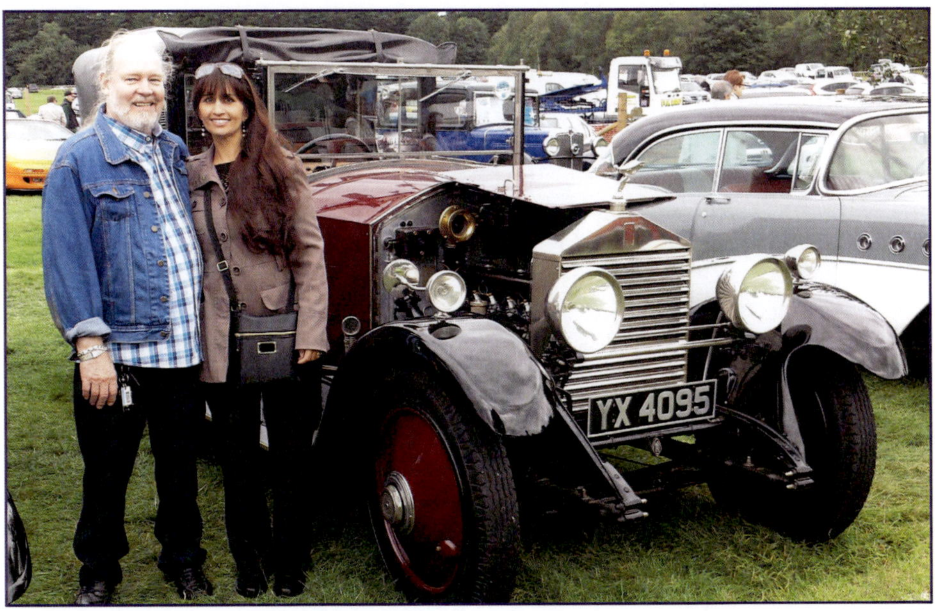

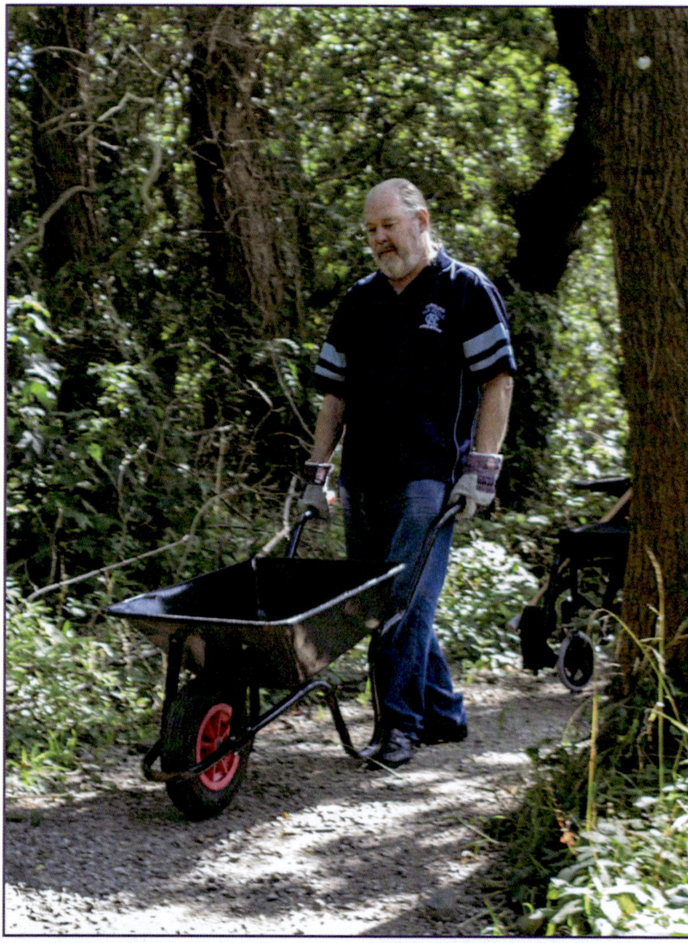

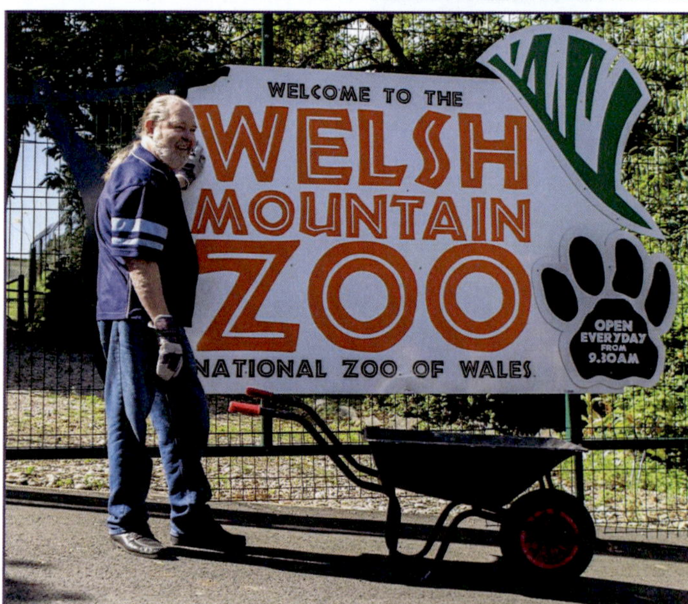
WELCOME TO THE
WELSH
MOUNTAIN
ZOO
NATIONAL ZOO OF WALES
OPEN
EVERYDAY
FROM
9.30AM

Chapter 10

MARTIN'S WHEELBARROW CHALLENGE

When Martin talked about his bucket list, he was tinkering away in the garage and he looked at many things and said, 'Well, I won't be needing this anymore, nor this, nor that, in fact none of these things.' He then looked at the wheelbarrow in the garage and asked Phil next door if he needed it up at his farm. Phil said, 'No, we are ok, thanks Martin.' Then our son Charlie came and said, 'Hey Dad, we could probably do with it up at our Welsh Mountain Zoo.' This was where Charlie worked. He said he would check with them and take it up.

Now Martin's mind went into thinking mode again. He said, 'Hey Wifey, I got an idea; you know we talked about raising awareness for this nasty cancer...what do you think about this? I will donate my wheelbarrow to the zoo and take it myself. We can get a little write-up in the local paper and it will be a little effort on my part to do something to get people to know the seriousness of this cancer and be more aware of it. You can do a great write-up and get it to the paper, because you are good at all that stuff.'

I was touched by Martin's idea and said, 'Martin, that's brilliant darlin' but have you forgot something? You are struggling to walk around the house and going upstairs. The zoo is just over a mile and a half, how will you cope?'

He said, 'We will manage. I got you by my side and if it kills me, at least I will die knowing I was doing something good in raising awareness to help someone else to not have to go through this tough time.'

Charlie came back to us to say that the zoo was happy to have the wheelbarrow and support us in our campaign for the awareness too. So we set the date and started planning the best way to make this happen. I asked Martin's cousin Andrew Stone if he could take some pictures en route to capture the story and a memory that we could treasure of our Martin.

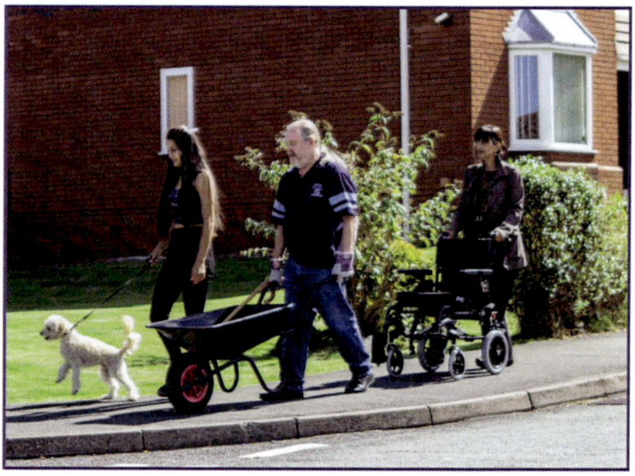

The wheelbarrow challenge was on. We filmed Martin bringing the wheelbarrow out of the garage and he got ready with his gardening gloves on. Picture this folks: we had our daughter Jennah leading the way with Buddy our dog. She wanted to be with her dad all the way. I had Martin's wheelchair ready just in case he felt too frail and couldn't manage the whole journey. Andrew had his camera all set ready to go and we took a deep breath and Martin and I said, 'Ok, let's do this.' And off we started the walk.

We also had a few of our dear friends: Maggie and Roy Jenkins, Jennifer and Tony Wetherill who rang to say they were making their way up to the zoo to support us. They all had health challenges of their own and couldn't walk the whole way but wanted to meet and cheer Martin at the 'finish line' when he delivered the wheelbarrow. Andrew took many pictures along the way and we had some of the neighbours looking to see what was going on. En route, we shared our situation and talked about the awareness campaign, which they were all so proud of Martin for doing this. It motivated Martin to know people appreciated his reasons and efforts.

Martin was very well-known in our community and the local school, where our kids went. When we used to get snowed in, parents who got stuck coming up the big hill to pick up the kids from school would get help from Martin. He would taxi the parents and children in the difficult conditions in his 4 x 4 vehicle. It was never any trouble for him to do this. The parents often said he should put in for being a school Governor for all that he did. I remember Martin telling me about an incident when he was waiting for one of our children outside an orthodontist appointment and noticed this guy park his car with a trailer a bit further up the hill. Martin noticed the trailer coming loose from the car and started rolling back. He ran towards it and stopped it. The man came out and realised what had happened and he couldn't thank Martin enough for that good deed. He said, 'Oh my God, imagine if my trailer had hit someone or caused a road accident.'

He was grateful for Martin being there to stop anything terrible happening. Even our children's friends always came to Martin for help with their broken bicycles, scooters and later their cars. They used to say to our kids, 'Your dad's cool, helping us out.' He always solved the problems. He was known as 'Daddy Cool'. Everyone had so much respect for Martin, for who was and what he did to help anyone anytime.

Back to our walk…Martin started to get a little tired and wanted a little sit down. I realised in all the running around I forgot to take some water for Martin to have on the walk. I rushed to our local shop and got a couple of bottles. Martin sat and gulped some water and was very grateful for the stop and the hydration. Then we carried on and walked through the woods with a little stop and breather before carrying on again. We were joined by our friend Maggie at the woods who had a beautiful beaming smile for Martin and said she was so proud of what he was doing. She said that her husband was waiting at the entrance of the zoo.

We had another corner of the walk to do which was a little incline and I could see that Martin was getting very tired. He said, 'We are nearly there, let's keep going, we can do this.' As we climbed this little hill, he said, 'Wait I need a rest.' He added, 'Most of the walk has been ok, but this little hill is a struggle. I don't know if the cancer will kill me but this hill is certainly challenging me.'

Whilst he had stopped by the post, I looked up and said, 'Hey Martin, look at the sign up above you.'

He looked at it and said, 'You're not funny, Wifey.' It was a disabled/elderly sign. Although he smiled and saw the funny side of it too. Martin was a very witty and cheeky guy, which was one of the most loveable things about him. He would always make me smile, laugh and blush. It was one of the characteristics of him that I was drawn to.

We were nearly there. I said, 'Martin, our Charlie is there. I can see him and Roy, Tony and Jennifer. They are there waiting for us.' Martin could see we were definitely almost there and bravely carried on. Then Charlie said in his cheeky way, knowing it would amuse Martin, 'Come on Dad, what's taking you so bloody long?'

Martin replied, 'This bloody hill is!' and laughed and called him a cheeky monkey.

Well, Martin made it to the entrance and everybody cheered him and said, 'Yay, well done Martin, you did it!' The head gardener was ready on the inside of the zoo gates and Martin proudly took his wheelbarrow and handed it over to Alan and they shook hands. It was such a lovely scene and I couldn't have been more proud of Martin in completing this task. He was determined to do it all by himself, with all his strength, courage and bravery and knowing the mission was to stay strong and fight it.

The wheelbarrow challenge was a success. My job was left to do the write-up on it, which I diarised to do and get in the local paper in due course. All Martin said after all that was, 'What I need now is a nice cup of tea and to put my feet up because I am shattered.' Our friends Roy and Maggie Jenkins drove Martin and I home and that's exactly what I did for Martin: make him that longed-for cuppa and we had a sit down and rest.

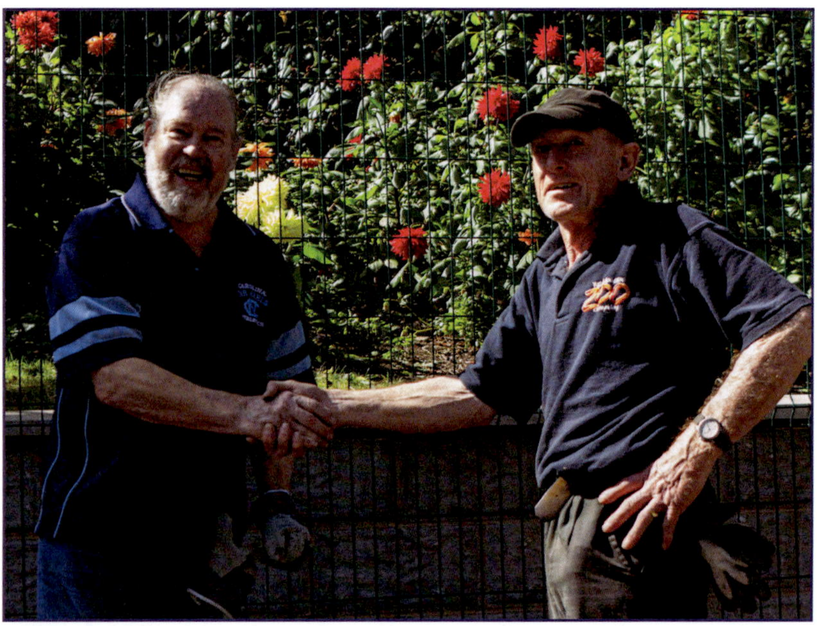

Chapter 11
CREATING FAMILY MEMORIES

Orme Photoshoot

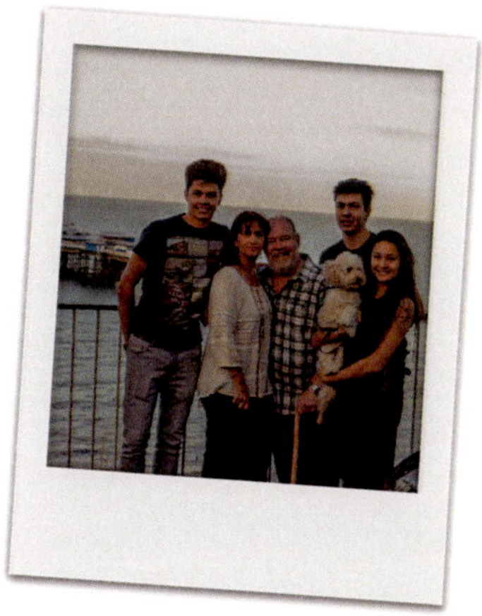

Another moment that I wanted was to capture some pictures of Martin on the Great Orme in Llandudno. This was one of the first holidays we spent when we were newly married and it seemed apt to capture some then and now memories. I asked the kids to come so we could have a few family pictures too. Some pictures of the children individually with their dad I thought would be nice for them to look back on over the years.

We were very grateful to our cousin Andrew once again agreeing to do these for us. It was also nice for him to have some time with his cousin too. Andrew's mum Nelly was the little sister of Martin's mum Lily. He was more than happy to capture these important memory-making pictures.

Mikyle drove up in the Peugeot that his dad gave him and the car that his dad taught him to drive in and I went in the Sonata that Martin bought me when he exchanged his 420 SEC Mercedes. We even had pictures taken of these cars because they had a lot to do with Martin's kind heart and a sign of always doing things to support and make his family happy. We had pictures taken by the summit, the panoramic view on top of the Great Orme with the North Wales coastline behind us and then by Llandudno Pier and the Happy Valley, where we brought our kids for treasure hunts and fun times.

We then finished the last few pictures by the paddling pool, near where we lived in Craig-y-Don. One of the funny pictures was when our grown-up children went to the park by the pool and climbed on the swings, slides and roundabout. Martin and I stood hand in hand and Martin whispered to me, 'We did all right, didn't we? Bringing up our kids in this wonderful way. Look at them all grown up and adults in their own way, thinking for themselves, doing things for themselves, all so independent. Our duty as parents has been done very well, I feel.'

I replied saying, 'Martin, I couldn't agree more, we did well. We are so proud of them and I'm proud of us. There was everyone thinking it wouldn't work.' It was a lovely reflection on the life that we made and the happiness we found within it.

Jennah's Birthday

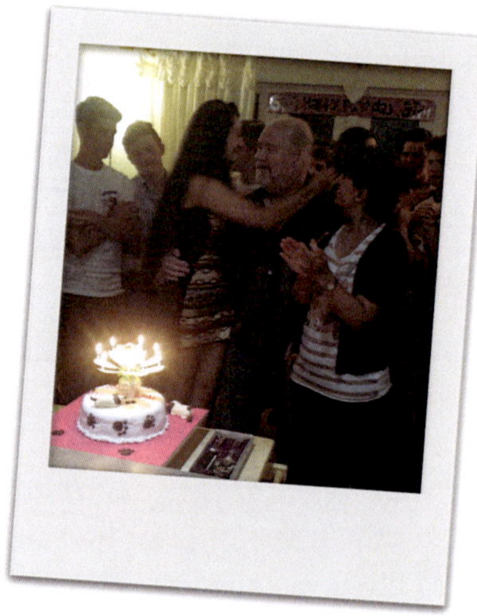

Now this birthday was not only a special year for celebration for our daughter Jennah, but it had another special meaning to it.

Jennah always said as a young child, 'When I am 16-years-old, I want this song playing on my birthday.' The song was: 'Sweet Sixteen' by Neil Sedaka.

At first Jennah wanted to book somewhere like a hotel or even our local community hall to accommodate lots of her friends to come to her special birthday party, but then realised that her dad would not be able to attend because of being on chemo and needing to stay away from lots of people with the risk of picking up any viruses or bugs. More important to her was having her dad there on her birthday with the painful truth that this may be the last birthday she would have with her dad. It was a sad thought on an occasion that is a celebratory in normal circumstances.

So, I suggested we have it at the house where her friends could use the kitchen area, conservatory and the garden, whilst leaving her dad undisturbed in the lounge. She was happy with that and we planned to get the party all set up. Glenys, my bestie decided to make her a special cake as she has done for us all in the years we've known her. I got the house decorated for a party mood. Jennah's friends were all made aware of her dad's health issues and were respectful about it. So immediate family and friends gathered to start the party and there was a lovely happy atmosphere. Jennah laughed and joked with all her friends and it was lovely to see everyone having a great time.

Then it was time to light the cake and Jennah wanted her dad to be there when she blew out the candles and asked me to get the special 'Sweet Sixteen' song to play as we lit the cake. Then suddenly everything changed. As soon as Jennah blew her candles on the cake, she turned to her dad and hugged him tight and sobbed on his shoulders. The reality of this painful truth hit us all in the room: this would be her last birthday with her dad being there to hug her. Nearly everyone was in tears. Martin was also so sad but kept his composure in front of everyone and slowly walked back to the lounge leaving the youngsters to continue the party. Jennah ran out to the garden to really let her tears flow and was comforted by her friends.

I went in to see if Martin was ok and he looked so sad but smiled and said, 'Yes I am ok, so sorry that this has put a dampener on the party.'

I said, 'Don't be so daft. Sadly this is the truth and a painful truth at that.' I went back to check on everyone else and unfortunately the mood of the party was just like bursting the balloon and her friends Rebecca and Conner started helping wrap up the evening by tidying up the mess and cleaning up everywhere. Two of Jennah's friends came over to me individually and asked for a small favour. They wanted to know if they could go in to say a hello personally to Martin, in case they didn't see him again. So I checked with Martin if he was ok with that and he said it was fine. Connor went in to say hi and chatted a little with Martin and shook his hand and thanked him for being who he was and said goodbye. Then Rebecca went in and she couldn't help but cry knowing that Martin would not be around much longer. She asked if she could give him a hug goodbye and he agreed. There were so many tears shed at this time. Martin was feeling the children's hurt and tried to keep a brave face on for them. How he could do that, I will never know because it was killing me – all the sadness around our family's situation.

The children all left respectfully and we had a little family time together and wound down the evening which was filled with such a range of emotions: fun, laughter, emotion, tears and special moments. Memories captured to live with us forever.

Even now when the Sweet Sixteen song is played anywhere, we all burst into tears as it brings everything all back.

Grandson James's 21st

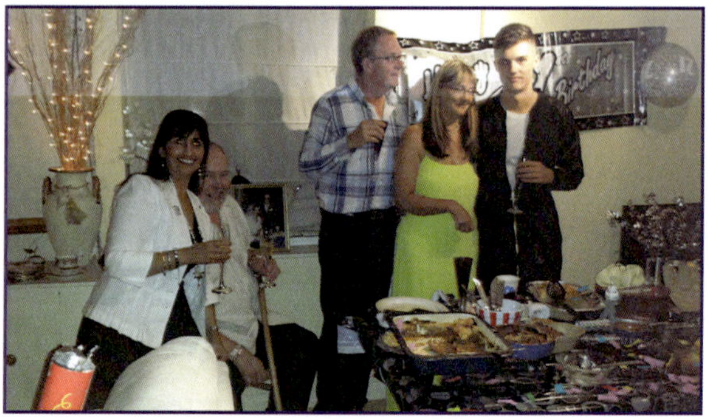

After the car show, we headed out to Martin's daughter Jacky and son-in-law Steve's house to celebrate Martin's grandson James's 21st Birthday. They all waited until we got there. Bless Martin, it was a heavy-going weekend but he stayed strong to deal with it all. He loved going to see Jacky and Steve, especially when Steve and Martin used to go off for a few drinks and lots of chit chats and come back all merry.

Steve and Martin were known as best drinking buddies. It was always so funny when they came back; they were a comedy duo. I remember when they were at our house and they came back in a merry way and started Mum's mobility scooter. It was like a comedy sketch. Martin told Steve the scooter drives well and then Steve said, 'Let's go round the block.' Then he ran off with the key and Jacky and I were trying to stop them messing about with the scooter. Steve said, 'Quick Martin, I got hold of Ghazala, you take the key and go. I got your back.' But little did he know that Jacky was quicker than him. She grabbed the key and ran upstairs and they no longer could run away with the scooter. They felt all their fun was taken away from them. It was one of the funniest scenes, where families just have some good fun and lots of humour and cheekiness. The kids would just watch us adults being like kids for a bit and we felt like the kids were the parents. There were so many funny stories of Steve and Martin and their times out.

At the party, Martin's grandchildren were so pleased that their grandad made it to James's birthday party and that he was well enough to be there. It was a great family party and more pictures of moments we knew we would look back on with great fondness.

Before the night was over, we all agreed to go to Chester Zoo together and as Charlie our son worked at Welsh Mountain Zoo and Chester Zoo was part of it , he said he would get us a family ticket and we planned to go in a fortnight's time, giving Martin some rest time too. Especially for his pending radiotherapy. We wanted to make sure he was well enough to handle it.

Family Day at Chester Zoo

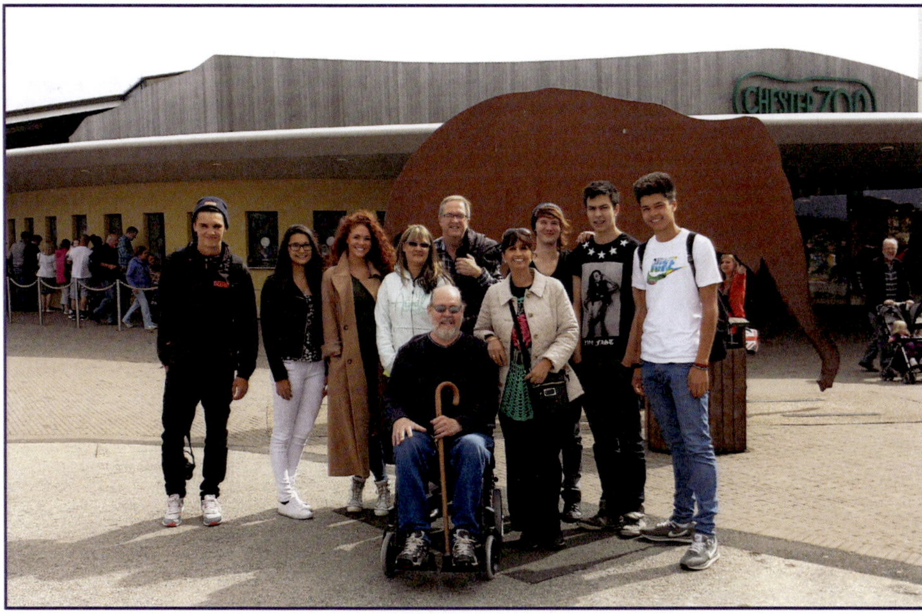

From one zoo to another, one of the things we had planned was for Martin to spend the time with his immediate family at Chester Zoo. This consisted of our three children, Mikyle, Charlie, Jennah, his eldest daughter Jacky, his son-in-law Steve, his grandchildren Adam, Stephanie and James and of course myself. I packed the car with his wheelchair and we all met at the entrance. Charlie organised the entrance ticket for the whole family and off we went around the different parts of the zoo. James, Martin's youngest grandson, brought his professional camera to capture some lovely pictures of the special family time too. Martin was delighted and had a beaming smile on his face seeing his family showing their unconditional love and attention for him. In particular they were doing their best to make his last days as wonderful as could be.

We laughed at the cheeky monkeys; we were impressed with the elephants' set up, we walked up to the deer and Martin said jokingly, 'Hey Wifey, there is your other family.' (my name Ghazala means a gazelle).

I laughed and said, 'Yes they are all here, too.' The meerkats were cute but we were not sure about the porcupine; he seemed a bit lost in there with them. The rhinos didn't do much but we got to see them. Then we all sat and had some lunch and I had Martin's medicine ready for him to take with the meal. He was on a high dose of Creon tablets as well as a few other things but the Creon was to help him digest the food because the pancreas had failed.

Then we continued to see all the other fascinating animals and had mid-afternoon ice cream. Martin loved his ice cream sundaes and truly tucked into it. One of the animals Martin was most impressed with was the graceful giraffes. He watched them in awe. He didn't like seeing animals in captivity but felt it was the only way we could see different species. He was happy that the animals were well looked after.

It's been a long time since I went to a zoo and I am glad I was here to have seen this and even more with my family. He was truly grateful and cherished every moment. It was cherished by us too having had this day with a man we all loved to bits. We then finished our day with a cup of tea and hugged each other as we all went our separate ways to our homes. It was a beautiful time spent with family.

Chapter 12
BACK TO HOSPITAL...

Martin had been on steroids and you could see he had put on some weight but had been coping with the radiotherapy quite well. When he went back to see the Oncologist on his weekly appointments, he asked when they would be starting on chemotherapy. The Oncologist said, 'We need to make sure that you are strong enough to cope with it after radiotherapy.'

Martin said, 'Yes but the cancer may be shrinking in the brain but it could be getting worse in the pancreas and other areas where it is at, so that might defeat the purpose.' The Oncologist insisted on doing all the tests to make sure that Martin was well enough to cope.

After the tests, the Oncologist confirmed that he was happy for Martin to be on chemo and the process started by getting what they call a picc line that was fitted into Martin's body which fed the regular dosage of the chemo drug. There were also plans put in place for the district nurses to come in to deal with the dressings and keep a note of his blood pressure, temperature, blood glucose levels etc, and the results were all being recorded on every visit. Martin was such a good patient, so calm and accommodating the necessary treatments, without any real questions, trusting the people and the process. I was also given instructions as to how to monitor the readings and do some tests. I felt like Martin's Nurse Jabeen on 24-hour call out. We had to be careful that Martin didn't get any infections with a temperature rise or other alerts.

I managed to handle the care for Martin very well and stayed as optimistic as could be knowing that his every day health was being monitored by the hospital, district nurses and by me his 'little wifey'.

Martin's health was getting worse and he was getting weaker. He had district nurses coming every day to sort his picc line and check his blood temperature and sugar levels and I continued to do follow on as well, recording everything. We would compare notes to see how things were being monitored and to keep an eye on anything unusual in the readings.

Martin was also a man that took great pride in his self-care, hygiene and how well he looked but even to brush his own hair was becoming very difficult for him. He always knew that I would step in when he could no longer manage and until that time, he wanted to keep his independence. One day he said, 'Ok Wifey, I need your help now.' I started to help by brushing his hair. He always had a great head of hair, which I used to describe as a lion's mane. Through the illnesses he used to wear it in a pony tail, which became his new look. This was now a very difficult time for a very proud man to be asking for help on these simple little things. As a husband and wife team we worked very well together with all the challenges life had thrown at us. As I took the brush and started to run it through Martin's hair, there were clumps falling out onto the brush. I was becoming very scared and even more worried. I was so gentle at brushing his hair too, but it still came out. He even asked me if it was coming out much, to which I said, 'Not a lot, you will be ok, don't worry.'

When I finished helping him freshen up, I went back to our bedroom and sat on the edge of the bed, whilst Martin stayed in the bathroom and rested a bit on the stool. I cried so much but as soon as I heard Martin coming back to the bedroom, I wiped my tears and looked at his kind, caring face and said, 'Martin how are you feeling, I mean really feeling?'

He sat by my side and said, 'Shall I tell you the truth? I am not ready to leave. I don't ever want to leave you and can't bear the thought of leaving you and the kids, ever.' He continued and said, 'I am going to change your world.' I looked at him in surprise, thinking he has only got weeks to live and he says he's going to change my world. I said, 'How?'

He replied, 'You'll see.' And that was as far as the conversation went.

By now Martin was struggling to get up and down the stairs and we talked about installing another stair lift back in the house, after we had Mum's taken out only a few months ago. I contacted the Macmillan nursing team and they said that there were some emergency grants that we could access to help make the necessary adaptations to help cancer patients for their care at home.

So, I started the process of finding a grant to help us pay for a stair lift. Unfortunately, it wasn't needed.

Martin - 'Wifey, I wish I was as brave as you.'
Ghazala - 'Martin I wish I was as clever as you.'

We always looked up to each other with the utmost respect.

Chapter 13
THE LAST WEEK

On Friday the 3rd of October, the stair lift people came to measure up the stairs and Martin for the lift. Shortly after, the nurse came to do her usual readings and recordings and then she said, 'Martin's temperature is high and we need to get him to hospital today to make sure he hadn't got an infection.' Last time when his temperature was up, he had a sinus infection and we had a bit of a problem at the lack of help and understanding at Glan Clwyd Hospital. They made so many errors and left us in the waiting room for ages. Even when putting the cannula in Martin's hand to take bloods, they seemed to have rushed it because the blood went everywhere and on the floor. They didn't even clear it up, even after asking them to do it, so I ended up wiping it off the floor.

Following the advice of the nurse about Martin's temperature being up, I phoned the Enfys Ward at the cancer centre of Glan Clwyd Hospital, explaining the situation and they suggested I bring Martin in to the hospital with an overnight bag too. Martin was not happy about the overnight bit, saying he didn't want to stay in the hospital. He said, 'Mum said the last time she went in that she wouldn't come out alive. I know I am dying, but I'm not ready for all that just yet.'

I said, 'We will tell them, but I will take something with us just in case. We need to get you seen. That's the most important bit.' We got ready and off we went.

When we arrived, the nurses did all the necessary tests and said to wait until the doctor arrived. I mentioned to the nurse that we were not keen on Martin staying in the hospital and any care that was needed we could do at home. She said that because the temperature was high and he needed intravenous antibiotics, he would need to be in hospital. She added, 'We don't really have any beds anyway so hopefully you may be able to go home. However, only the doctor can decide that for you.'

When the doctor eventually came to see Martin, he read the notes, asked some questions and then he said, 'Based on the tests and your vital statistics, we need to keep you in and start you straight away on intravenous antibiotics.' This was something we did not want to hear but had to be realistic and knew that Martin could get worse. Then we would blame ourselves for not listening to the professionals and agreed to have Martin stay. They then had to try and find a bed for him and we had to sit in the waiting area until they called us in to say everything was all set up.

We eventually got taken to the ward where there was a bed ready for Martin and he was set up on antibiotic drip. I sat on the chair by his side and then the doctor came and said they were doing some other paperwork and looking at the plan they were going to put him on. When he came back a little later, he pulled the curtain around the bed and sat down to talk to us with a serious look on his face and some paperwork for us to sign. He said, 'We don't have a CPR (Cardiopulmonary Resuscitation) form filled in for you on file.' We both looked at each other in shock and I turned to the doctor and said, 'CPR? Why do we need to have that at this stage? We came in with Martin having a high temperature, but you are making it sound like his death could be imminent.'

He said, 'There are drugs we need to give to Martin and we need to cover any emergency situation in the event it arises.' I asked the doctor to leave us alone for a minute while we talked to each other. When the doctor left, Martin said, 'Hey Wifey, maybe my time is up sooner that we thought.'

I turned to him and said, 'Oh stop it, that is not the case. They have to do all this admin as standard protocol.' So, after a little set back from that decision-making exercise, we eventually decided to sign the necessary documents and allow the necessary steps to be taken in the event of an emergency situation. I stayed with Martin as late as I could and promised him I would get there as early as possible in the morning.

When I came home, I realised that our kids had sorted their own dinner and looked after the house whilst I was at the hospital, but they were very worried about their dad. I said, 'Your dad is doing ok and I will take you guys to see him tomorrow.'

When I arrived at the hospital on the Saturday morning it was breakfast time.

Martin sat there and said, 'I didn't sleep well with so much noise and machines bleeping and being worried about what is actually happening to me.' He said he didn't want to eat anything either. I tried to help encourage him to eat a little bit, but he said he couldn't face eating anything. Martin was on Creon tablets and I noticed that he only had one tablet, which was half of the dose prescribed. So, I asked the nurse if Martin's medicine had been changed and she said that is what he has to take. I argued the point and asked her to show me his medicine card to see for myself. When she unlocked the bedside cabinet and we both looked, she realised I was right, and she apologised for the oversight and promised to make sure that it didn't happen again.

I stayed with Martin chatting for a bit then I was asked to sit in the 'quiet room' whilst they freshened him up and made the beds for the day. Whilst sitting in the quiet room, I was reflecting on how things were moving fast and out of my control. All these medical people seemed to have taken over and I felt somewhat helpless in taking care of my man. It was like it was all in the hands of God and it frightened me a lot wondering what I should do or could do to help Martin get better.

Then I got a call from my best friend Glenys, asking how Martin was doing. I gave her an update and shared my concerns with her. I also asked her if she wanted to come and say hi to Martin. She said she would love to, if it was ok to do so. I checked with the staff and they said it was fine. She came after lunchtime. She slowly went over to Martin and quietly said, 'How are you Martin?' He looked at her and smiled.

I could tell he was pleased to see her but did not say too much other than, 'Well, at least you've come to see me this time unlike last time.'
She said, 'I did come last time Martin, when you told us all to leave your bedside.'
'What, you came then, did you? Oh I don't remember that,' he said.
I said, 'Martin you asked the whole family to leave.'
He replied, 'Then I am sorry, Glenys.'
She said, 'It's ok Martin, you don't need to apologise, you were very poorly.'

We sat and talked a little bit more and then the nurse came to do Martin's medications and asked Glenys if she could wait in the quiet room. Shortly after the nurse finished, I went to invite Glenys back and went to the quiet room, only I couldn't see her in there. All I saw was nurses having their tea break and cakes. I kept looking around and saw Glenys was stood outside in the corridor of the Enfys Ward. I asked her why she was there and she said, 'I was asked to leave because it was the staff tea break.' I couldn't believe I was hearing this because the staff had a dedicated room for their breaks and the quiet room was supposed to be for visitors and their family and friends. I made a mental note of this to speak to someone about it. It was wrong that the staff were taking advantage of it.

Later in the evening our children came and Martin was so pleased to see them too. I took a picture of the happy little scene. Charlie started telling his dad about his MG's carburetor problems and Mikyle started telling him about his car and they just loved talking to their dad about cars. Martin loved to help them understand the cars better. Jennah chatted about Buddy our dog and Tizzy and Sushi our cats. They were also aware that they didn't want to tire their dad too much and they hugged him and told him they loved him very much and that he would be all right and then they went home. I stayed until very late and left about 11pm.

The following day Jacky, Steve and his grandson came over to see him and chatted for a bit. Once again the family were aware not to tire Martin especially as he wasn't talking too much and looked very tired. They hugged him and said goodbye and left.

Martin felt like he was struggling to breathe and certainly didn't feel like eating any food at all. He also developed a high temperature; the nurses were saying that his CRP levels were very high. They got some oxygen for him too. I felt I needed him to rest up and decided to leave earlier than normal.

Then on Monday I was there early and to make sure Martin had his breakfast. I noticed there was only one Creon capsule on his tray. I asked the nurse the same question and they said sorry and said they would double-check it. I asked to speak to a senior nurse who would be more responsible in taking action. They took my message and said they would pass it on. I sat and waited and waited but nobody came to me. This gave me little confidence in the staff, as there seemed to be so many errors being made and patients' care not being administered properly. Going back to Martin, he was struggling to breathe and they said they wanted to do an x-ray and were preparing the necessary arrangements for wheelchair and the paperwork to get Martin down to x-ray room. I went with him and then when we got back, one of the doctors came to see us. They said that Martin had fluid on the lungs and they needed to add more medication to help with that. It was one of the reasons he was struggling to breathe. So that was all put in place.

On Monday, Martin looked worse, he was sweating terribly and his CRP levels were concerning. This was explained to Martin and he was getting worried of what to expect next. For us we could tell he was taking a turn for the worse. Martin then asked me to ask if Jennah could charge his phone and could I bring today's newspaper with me when I came back with the kids. I was a little confused at his request but agreed to do it.

The phone was charged and the kids had brought the Daily Mail, Martin's favourite newspaper. As they sat by Martin's side, Martin asked me to close the curtains around his bed. He asked me to go round and sit by his other side and held my hand and asked Jennah to record a video on the phone. We were very concerned about what he was trying to say and do but respected his wishes.

Then he said, 'As you all know, my condition is getting worse and my breathing is very bad and I am not sure if I will make it out alive. In the event I don't, I wanted to do my last will and testament, because that is something I never got to do and all I wanted to do was everything I could to protect you all and sort things out before I go.' This was so sad to hear and deal with. It turns out he wanted the newspaper so he could prove the date of the recording.

Upon Martin's instructions, Jennah started to record the video on the phone and Martin spoke his words and wishes about leaving everything he had (which he kept apologising for that it wasn't much) to me and to help with the house, the children's education and all our futures. Part way through the filming, Jennah started to cry as all this was upsetting her so much. Her young broken-heart couldn't cope seeing her dad in this terribly poorly way and yet he was more bothered about our welfare than his own health. She handed the phone to Charlie to continue with the recording. As you can imagine, it was a very difficult, sensitive and heart-breaking situation but we knew we had to stay strong for Martin and go through it. As much as I wanted to console the children, Martin had a grip of my hand and I wanted to cry myself.

After the recording, we all hugged each other and there was so much love shared through our tears at this difficult time. The kids left shortly after as Martin was so tired and kept sleeping. Once again, I stayed as long as I needed to. Then just near midnight, when Martin had settled to sleep, I went up to the nurses' station and told them to call me if Martin was needing me at any time in the night.

Then when I went back in the morning on Tuesday, Martin said once again he couldn't eat much and was in a bad way with his breathing and couldn't sleep. I said they were told to call me but they hadn't. He said he couldn't even get to call them because the buzzer was out of reach. I raised this issue with them too and they took note. By now, I didn't have much confidence with them that this was even going to be addressed.

Martin's eldest grandson Adam wanted to come and see his grandad at the hospital. We were told that family could come anytime. So, he greeted his grandson with a hug and had a brief chat, but Adam knew that his grandad was too weak to talk much. This really upset him that his grandad had deteriorated this much and said to me that he was going to go to the quiet room for a bit. He went and I stayed with Martin. Shortly after, I went to see if Adam was all right and saw that he was not in the quiet room. Like Glenys, he was in the corridor and I asked him why he was not in the quiet room. He said the staff asked him to leave as they were having their tea break. He and I stood in the corridor in tears. We were by the lift where everyone was coming and going so we couldn't even cry in private. It was a terrible situation and we were not impressed with some of the staff at Enfys Ward at the cancer centre of Bodelwyddan Hospital. We felt their lack of care and support during this seriously upsetting time.

On Wednesday, the rest of the family came to visit, including Martin's children and grandchildren. They wanted to spend some extra time with Martin and keep his spirits uplifted. Unfortunately, I had my Bollywood classes to teach and didn't want to leave, but Martin said, 'You go. At least I have Jacky and the kids here and I will see you when you've finished.' So I left them and went to teach.

Charlie said to me afterwards that his dad was a bit chattier and even laughed with them all. He said, 'I was having a cheeky banter with Dad about the car and things and he said jokingly: *Oh piss off, Charlie* in a fun, light-hearted way.' It made everyone laugh knowing that Martin was in a better mood. I was pleased to know that the family had had some nice time together.

When I finished my class, I was exhausted from a back-to-back cardio fitness workout and feeling very hungry. I grabbed a quick bite to eat en route to the hospital. When I got there, I saw that Martin was resting nicely. He said it was lovely to have all the children chatting away with him earlier. However, he was tired now and wanted to sleep. I didn't say too much to him, but just sat by his side and held his hand. Then after a while I said, 'I will let you sleep now, Martin and go home but will be back in the morning.' He didn't want me to go. He said my being with him gave him comfort and the staff didn't really check much or they didn't come quickly when the buzzer was pressed. So, I stayed a bit longer, but I couldn't stay the night as it was an open ward with 3 other patients there. Finally Martin was ok for me to go. I reassured him that if he needed me to let them know and I would drive back. I spoke to one of the nurses and said it was important. Martin seemed a little worried and didn't want me to leave, so please could they make sure they called me if he seemed unsettled at any time in the night. They made a note on the file and then I left going home with an uneasy feeling.

While I was going out of the hospital, I had a message from my friend Cathy (and one of my Bollywood dancers). She said she had a card for Martin and was going to come and see him but wasn't sure when would be an ok time to do so to hand it to him. I told Cathy that Martin was not up to any visitors other than immediate family and that his condition was getting worse. We agreed to meet in the car park of the hospital, as her friend who was having a baby had gone to hospital and she was accompanying her. She gave me a card to give Martin and to tell him she was thinking of him and sending her best wishes.

Just after midnight before I settled down to sleep, I phoned the hospital to see if Martin was all right, so I could go to sleep rest assured. They said he was but due to his breathlessness they had to give him maximum oxygen and he was settled. I said ok, but to please let me know if I needed to come in and the nurse said she would.

On Thursday morning, I called the hospital to say I was on my way and to ask if Martin was ok and if he needed me to bring him anything in particular. The nurse said that Martin was stable but he had had a bit of an accident in the night. I couldn't believe what I was hearing. I said, 'What kind of accident and why did someone not phone me?' She couldn't answer that question as to why nobody called me. She said she had not long been on her day shift. I said I would be up to the hospital straight away. On my way, I was thinking all sorts of things. Had he wet the bed or got out of the bed and fell, or what? She had said they would explain when I got there.

On arrival, I went straight to his bed because there were no nurses on the reception. I asked Martin what had happened. He was trying to speak but was so breathless, he wasn't making much sense. He kept saying he couldn't breathe and felt like he was drowning. Then the two other patients on the ward next to him said that Martin had a panic attack and they realised he couldn't reach his buzzer so they called the staff with their buzzers. I couldn't believe what was happening. It had taken other terminally ill patients to have to do a call-out for the nurses for an emergency just because Martin couldn't reach the buzzer. A problem we had explained before. They then explained that there was blood everywhere on his bed because in the process of the panic attack, Martin had pulled the cannula out of his hand, which led to the bleeding. The nurses finally got there to tidy things up and sort Martin out. I was so angry and decided I was going to stay with him day and night and did not trust the staff at all. I had already decided that there were too many errors along the process and I would be making an official complaint, but right now I had to deal with Martin's best care.

When the nurse came to talk to me, she tried to explain what the other two patients had already explained to me. I made it my business to check Martin's record to see if he had had any change of medication etc... I also noticed that Martin's intravenous was empty and asked the nurse when she was changing it. She said after the breakfast round. I sat and waited for a while and I asked again and was told the senior nurse was on her way. I also told her that I was not going home at all now and how sad I was that this had happened. She said that Martin's Oncologist was coming round to see him at about 11am and I could raise these issues with him too.

Then mid-morning the Oncologist arrived with his secretary and sat by Martin's side with his file in his hands. He said, 'Martin, as you know, we had to take the picc line out and it was sent to the labs. We've had the results that there is some bacteria there.'

Martin asked him when they would put in another picc line. The Oncologist said, 'You are too weak at this point to even think about it. You've also had fluid on the lungs, hence the breathing issues, your CRP levels have been dangerously high and we will not be doing any further chemo whilst these things are happening. There isn't a lot more we need to intervene with right now but need to also instruct the Palliative Care team to take over now. We have decided that it is better we move you to your own private room and your wife can stay overnight too. We will make you as comfortable as possible but we will want you to continue taking the antibiotics.' He got up and said goodbye to Martin.

When he left, Martin looked at me and said, 'Well Wifey, it's c'est la vie time, I guess.' He continued with a disheartened voice. 'The Oncologist might as well have put a nail in the coffin with that meeting because he has literally closed the book on me. What hope does that give me? It's over.'

At that point I couldn't argue with Martin's comments or observation because I also felt they had said a 'final goodbye'. The Oncologist was Martin's last hope to turn things round at least for some extra time, which is what we both had wanted all along knowing Martin's condition was terminal. But it seemed they didn't want to do much more other than see the process to a close. I also went out to the nurse's station and asked why Martin's antibiotics hadn't been sorted and that it was now lunchtime. I was concerned the missed dose of this important medicine was once again not dealt with the priority that it needed.

When after lunch the senior nurse came, she asked me to sit in the quiet room, while she sorted Martin out. I sat in the quiet room and could see Martin from there. I noticed she changed the drip and went to reception and then went back to Martin then came to me and said, 'I believe you were concerned that Martin hadn't had his morning antibiotics? Well, I have checked his file and he has,' and then showed me the label that he had already had it. I asked, 'When did he have it?' And she said, 'After breakfast'. At this point I had to argue with her.

I said, 'He hasn't! I was here just before as I do come every morning to help Martin eat breakfast and it was to be changed and never was. I haven't left his side, not even to go to the ladies', so I know he didn't have it.'

She said, 'Here is the label and it's written in the file.'

I said, 'First off, I know the difference from the label that was on there before to the one you are showing me now and I don't know why they would write something in the file that they have given it when clearly they haven't.' Now, I didn't even believe the senior nurse in charge and I felt she was lying to me and I told her that I didn't believe any of it. They made me feel like I was lying. It was an awful situation to have to fight over the medication and there was Martin dying. I wouldn't want anyone to have to go through these awful situations as we all did. I also told her that Martin may have a terminal condition with his cancer but his head was still fully aware of what was or wasn't happening so to please give us some respect. She said she would look into it, but never came back to me on anything. It was like it was dismissed under the carpet.

Martin said their idea of putting me in another room was another indicator that it was time to say goodbye. Martin was dying but not daft. He knew what was happening. I tried to reassure him that I would take care of him no matter what was on the agenda. I said, 'When our number is up, our number is up and in the meantime we must stay strong. While they get the other room ready, I will go home and get some more t-shirts for you and a few bits and bobs for me to stay here with you and then we will settle you in there and I will be with you 24/7.' He just smiled at me knowing I would do my best with whatever was ahead of us.

I updated the children on what was happening and to make sure that they kept the conversations uplifted for their dad because he was fully aware of what was happening. Later, when I got back to the hospital, we got Martin moved to the private room and settled him down. The children came shortly after and Jennah took a picture of her dad in his room and she wrote his name on his whiteboard. Mikyle, Charlie, Jennah, Jamie (Jennah's boyfriend) and I had dinner with him. Jamie even dropped the dinner plate and startled Martin, but we had a chuckle on him. Martin enjoyed all of us eating together, although he couldn't eat much but for the sake of the children, he made an effort. The children felt a little happier that they had some quality time with their dad.

On Friday, I was chatting a little with Martin, whilst keeping an eye on the BP machine which was now recording 24/7. I remember Martin saying, 'Wifey, in the event I get worse and not fully with it, because I am now starting to feel very weak and very tired, please promise me you will help me keep my pride and dignity, especially in front of the family.' I gave Martin my word; he needn't worry about a thing. I had all that taken care of and made sure he was well looked after. He said, 'I do love you, Wifey.' And I replied, 'I love you too, darlin'.'

The children came over and Martin had asked Charlie to bring the papers for the carburetor, which he brought and wanted his dad to have a look. Sadly Martin's concentration level was very poor and he said, 'Charlie leave it there and I will look at them later.' Charlie was sad that his dad was not well enough to look at the papers of the work on the carburetor. Martin had also said to bring the laptop so he could let me know all the details of the files that he had and what to do with them. I told him I would get that for him tomorrow. Jacky came and so did his granddaughter Stephanie. We all talked nice and quietly knowing Martin just wanted calmness. When the children were going home, Stephanie knew she wouldn't be able to come over on the weekend and needed to say goodbye to her grandad. She knew she may not be able to see him alive again. She fought her tears and tried so hard to say bye but she struggled, because nobody wants to say goodbye to their loved one knowing it may be the last time. She gave him a hug and a kiss and went home in tears. It was really upsetting to see her like that. Then when they all went, the nurse came and settled Martin for the night.

On Saturday morning, one of the doctors came in to see Martin and checked the records and asked to speak to me in the quiet room. I went over and sat down. The quiet room always had a sad feeling with it because it had enough tissue boxes for all the tears that have been shed in there.

The doctor explained to me that Martin's time was limited and we could only but keep him as comfortable as possible and to prepare for the inevitable. Of course, I reached out for the tissues, and cried and didn't know how I was going to handle this situation. I said to the doctor that I wanted to know if I had time to go home and get some more t-shirts for Martin, because he was sweating so much and that I wouldn't be long and he said, 'You go. There is nothing more you can do. What will be will be and it's in the hands of God.' The way he said it, made me feel like he didn't have a heart, he was so cold and didn't really seem bothered about the importance of my needing to be phoned. He delivered the information that he needed to and then went. In the afternoon the palliative nurse came and introduced herself to Martin and asked if he needed any painkillers, to which he said he had no pain. They said they were on standby for anything he needed help with.

I stayed and cried for a bit then I went home, rushed around like crazy to get all the things I needed to get including the laptop that Martin wanted, had a quick 10-minute shower to freshen up in case I couldn't afterwards. I had no call from the hospital. However, I rushed back to be with Martin not knowing anything on timing. When I got there, he was still breathing and settled. I put everything down. Later in the afternoon Jacky, Steve, and our children came to see Martin. Whilst they were there chatting Martin had a little funny turn and started panicking to breathe and saying things like, 'Quickly, hurry up, I need to save my wife. We are drowning.' He wanted to get off the bed. I asked the family to leave. I had promised Martin I was going to respect his pride and dignity. So, the family went, the nurses came and arranged for palliative nurses to come too. They gave him an injection to settle his panic attack and before long Martin relaxed and went to sleep.

Later that evening, as I sat on the chair by Martin's side, I realised that we never got to open the laptop to do the stuff Martin wanted to, but I was more concerned that he was not in distress. It was getting near midnight and Martin had not moved much at all since his injection and I was getting anxious about the whole thing. I kept asking the nurses if he was still with us because he hadn't moved much at all. They kept assuring me that he was still alive and well but the medication had relaxed him and the rest was what he needed right now. They got me a drink of tea to help me settle myself and the nurse said I was tired and it was making me more anxious. She said that I must try and close my eyes for a bit too.

I sat praying to get some strength to deal with what I felt was the nearing of time to say goodbye. Then shortly after I got a phone call. It was my friend and one of my Bollywood dancers Jennifer. She said she was thinking about me and felt the urge to call me to see if I was coping all right and to see if there was anything she could do to help. Jennifer was studying her nursing course, so her natural need to care was to reach out to me at this difficult time. I said to her that I was worried about how to cope with this next hurdle and mentioned to her that Martin hadn't moved at all since his injection and I wasn't sure if he would ever wake up. I told her that we didn't get a chance to say goodbye or anything and I was hoping and praying he would wake up again. She did her best to listen to me and be with me at this time, which helped me a lot. I felt she was like an angel sent to comfort me during those last few hours.

Eventually I was getting tired and we said goodbye to each other on the phone and I shut my eyes for a little sleep.

I remember the machines were bleeping and noises from other patients going on and just so much activity during the night that I really didn't settle properly at all. The next thing I knew it was about 6.30 am and I remember a nurse came and said that Martin was sweating a lot and need to put a fresh dry sheet on for him and another pillowcase for him to be comfortable. She said she would be finishing the night shift and wanted to get him sorted for the next lot of nurses to take over. She said he was comfortable and his heart was beating ok. I said to her that he hadn't moved for over 12 hours and asked if that was normal. She said he was ok and stable and then left.

Martin was trying to talk, but he couldn't get his words out properly. I said:

'I know you're trying to tell me something Martin, but I can't figure out what it is, darling.'

Martin reached for my hand and took it in both of his hands and brought them to his heart. I realised he was trying to tell me that he loved me.

I shall never forget that precious moment, captured forever.

Chapter 14
THE FINAL GOODBYE

Sunday 12th October 2014

I remember getting washed and ready for the day. I went over to Martin and started talking to him. 'Hey Martin, come on wake up, you have been asleep for too long.' He twitched his fingers a little, so I continued talking. 'Come on Martin, there's sleeping and there's sleeping. What do you think you are, sleeping beauty? Please wake up and show me your blue eyes again.' Then suddenly, Martin started moving and was trying to open his eyes. I carried on talking, thinking he can hear me and this is good so I said, 'Yes you haven't looked into my brown eyes for ages and I need to see your beautiful blue eyes again. Let me know you can hear me Martin.' Then I was delighted when he actually opened his eyes and looked right at me. I said, 'Thank God you're awake.'

He was trying to talk but he couldn't get his words out properly. It was very mumbled up words so I said, 'I know you're trying to tell me something Martin, but I can't figure out what it is darling. Do you need something?' He pointed at the glass of water. I remember the nurse telling me not to let him sip the water from a glass, because he would have a swallowing difficulty but instead, try slowly wetting his lips with the sponge lollipop. I explained this to Martin and then followed through on the nurse's instruction. Then Martin reached for my hand and was trying to tell me something. He took my hand in both his hands and brought them to his heart. I realised he was trying to tell me that he loves me. My eyes filled with tears and I looked at him and I said, 'I love you too.' I hugged him so dearly. We had 'our little precious moment'. I told him that he would be fine and he just smiled at me. Shortly after, I phoned the children and asked them to come to the hospital as soon as they could because their dad was awake and they could talk to him. I had a feeling that this would probably be the last time they would be able to talk to him, because Martin could no longer talk. We only had a very small window to say whatever we needed to.

At about 8.30am, the children arrived and came straight into the room. I was just telling them that their dad woke up and was talking and then the nurses came in and asked us if we could give them about 5 minutes so they could change the bed sheets and freshen Martin for the day. I told her that the kids had just arrived so could we have ten minutes with Martin and then we would wait in the quiet room. She was adamant she had to get the sheets done, and insisted we come back as she would only be 5 minutes. We were not happy but we went into the quiet room and I decided to prepare the children to handle this situation with the best possible support from me. I asked them to go one by one into their dad's room and spend no more than 5-10 mins to tell their dad whatever they wanted to. Just to speak from their heart but keep the conversation light so it didn't upset their dad too much. I suggested the youngest of the children go first, which was of course our daughter Jennah then Charlie and then Mikyle.

The nurse came to us 20 minutes later and said we could go in now (which wasn't the 5 minutes she told us). Jennah got up and composed herself and went to her dad. She came back sobbing after ten minutes and sat on my lap and wept her heart out. I asked her if her dad was ok; she nodded at me. I then told Charlie to go in and reminded him not to talk too long and keep it light. I sat and tried to console Jennah and get Mikyle prepared to go after Charlie. I realised 10 minutes had gone by and got worried that Charlie was not back and wanted to make sure all was ok. I decided to go check. I asked Mikyle to come with me so he could speak to his dad, and then Charlie was just coming out also in tears. This really was breaking my heart seeing our children hurting so much but I continued to stay composed and strong for the children.

Mikyle said, 'What shall I say to Dad?' I told him to tell his dad whatever he felt and that he loved him and left him to his private time. After 10 minutes, I asked all of us to go in there. We had Jamie with us too who was additional support for Jennah, being her boyfriend.

We all stood by Martin and I watched his face looking so sad and he was struggling to breathe. I couldn't tell whether it was a breathing issue or if he was crying too. Whilst holding Martin's hand I said, 'Martin, please breathe slowly just as the nurse told you.' I gripped his hand and continued as the children stood by their dad and also grabbed his hand. I talked in a loving relaxed way saying, 'Hey Martin, it's ok we are right by you, Mikyle, Charlie, Jennah and Jamie are right here with you. Jacky and Steve are on their way and will be here anytime now. So just relax darling.' The next thing was, Martin struggled to breathe further and closed his eyes. I knew he had gone. Jennah screamed the loudest and ran out of the room. Jamie went after her to comfort her. Jennah went to cry in the quiet room but once again that room was not available to anyone because the staff were having their tea break. My daughter had just lost her dad and couldn't even have the privacy to cry in that room, instead she sat on the stairs by the hall in the corridor crying her heart out.

I stayed with our sons and we all hugged and cried together but in the process of hugging them, I got a terrible nose bleed that I couldn't stop. I was trying to support the children but was in so much distress too that my soulmate, my best friend, my life partner, my husband, the father of our children, had left this earth forever. It was so final. It felt like someone had ripped my heart out and I was not only hurting for my children but for my own loss too. It was so awful. We were all beside ourselves with our loss. The next thing I could hear was steps walking into the room and it was Jacky, Martin's eldest daughter with her husband Steve just behind her. As she walked in to a room full of us crying, Jacky looked at me and said, 'Has Dad gone?'

I replied, 'Only just, Jacky.' She went over towards the head of the bed and gently kissed her dad's forehead and said, 'Goodbye Dad.' I cannot explain how terribly sad our situation was losing our big man with a big heart leaving us with a big hole in our lives.

Shortly after, we were all escorted to a private room where the staff made us some tea. The family went but I stayed a little longer to take a moment. I felt numb and lost realising that suddenly our life had changed forever. With a heavy heart I walked out with one final look at Martin who lay there peacefully. As I arrived in the room with the family, I said to Jacky, 'Tell me this is not really happening; tell me your dad hasn't gone.'

She hugged me and said, 'Dad has gone.' I really didn't want to hear those words but knew it had happened.

We stayed a little bit longer until they sorted Martin's body for us to go in again. I did go back just to be sure that it was really happening. I opened the door and there was Martin, laying like he was fast asleep and at peace. We all walked out of the hospital with great sadness trying to console each other on the way to our cars. We followed each other in convoy back to our home.

I remember arriving at the house and knew walking through the front door that it would never be the same. As I stepped in the house, there was a sense of a cold and lonely feeling. We were all feeling like zombies, trying to comprehend what had just happened. I remember our neighbours Lexcie and Iain came across, as they had been with us through the journey. They had come to pay their condolences and offer some comfort to us. Steve helped out by making tea for us all but didn't realise that he was making Earl Grey tea, which was only ever used by me, so he had to do it over again with the normal tea. This gave us a little light-hearted distraction and a breather from our sadness. This reminded me of when Glenys once made a cup of tea for Martin and I and gave him Earl Grey tea by mistake and Martin nearly spat it out and said, 'What are you doing to me Glenys, killing me with tea?' He was definitely not a fan of Earl Grey, and used to say how can people drink this tea with fragrance. We had a a good chuckle on it and Glenys never made that mistake again. It was a little Martin reminder when Steve made that drink.

Afterwards, Jacky and Steve had agreed that we needed some time out and wanted us to go back to their house to switch off from everyone and have some privacy. We headed to their home in Cheshire for the night.

When we came back, we had to let everyone know about Martin's passing and do all the necessary official paperwork. I had to go back to the hospital to collect a few belongings and arrange to get the death certificate. The lady sorting that out for me asked if we were looked after during this time and if not, could she arrange an appointment to see the Oncologist. I said I was not at all happy with so many things and that I did want to raise my concerns, with the Oncologist or needed the details of the person I should address my concerns with. She set up a meeting with our Oncologist for the following Thursday.

I got Martin's death certificate and Mikyle went with me as we sorted these formalities. Then Charlie went with me to the appointment with the Oncologist's secretary. What was going to be about a 10 -15 minute meeting lasted about an hour explaining the problems encountered by us and my Martin as a patient. I could see he seemed surprised and a little taken aback. His secretary took many notes and they said they would investigate it all and let us know of their findings. I made sure I told them about the bed sheet changing episode and that they couldn't even respect our last little wish/request.

I was told later by the secretary that the reason they wanted to change the bed sheets was because Martin had soiled the bed. I told her that this was a lie. I said, 'How could they know the bed was soiled when they were in the corridor and came into the room determined to change the sheets without inspecting the patient or the bed, even after me telling them that the sheets were changed earlier on?' The secretary couldn't answer me back with anything else. I said that I would be taking this further. Some mistakes, I can deal with, after all we are all human – but liars, I cannot tolerate. She said she would take my feedback to them again.

There were too many situations, too many mistakes and too many bad excuses in my opinion and nobody really was taken to task. There had been no written confirmation about making these changes, in fact, it felt like it was all falling on deaf ears. It gave us little hope for other patients, who were not so vocal like me.

We lost two members of our family in this hospital and all they could say was sorry. Our life had been turned upside down, changed forever. We were also financially affected and it seemed nobody really understood the bad situation we were left in. Their 'sorry' was just an insult to injury and it was unforgivable in my view.

I had the opportunity to discuss this with our local Assembly Member, who referred me to Betsi Cadwalder Health Board. I made an appointment with them and went through all the details with tears in the meeting as this was difficult enough with what had happened, but felt I needed to voice my concerns. I knew it wasn't going to bring Martin or Mum back, but if it could help someone else so they didn't have to go through the same experience we did, then it would be worth it.

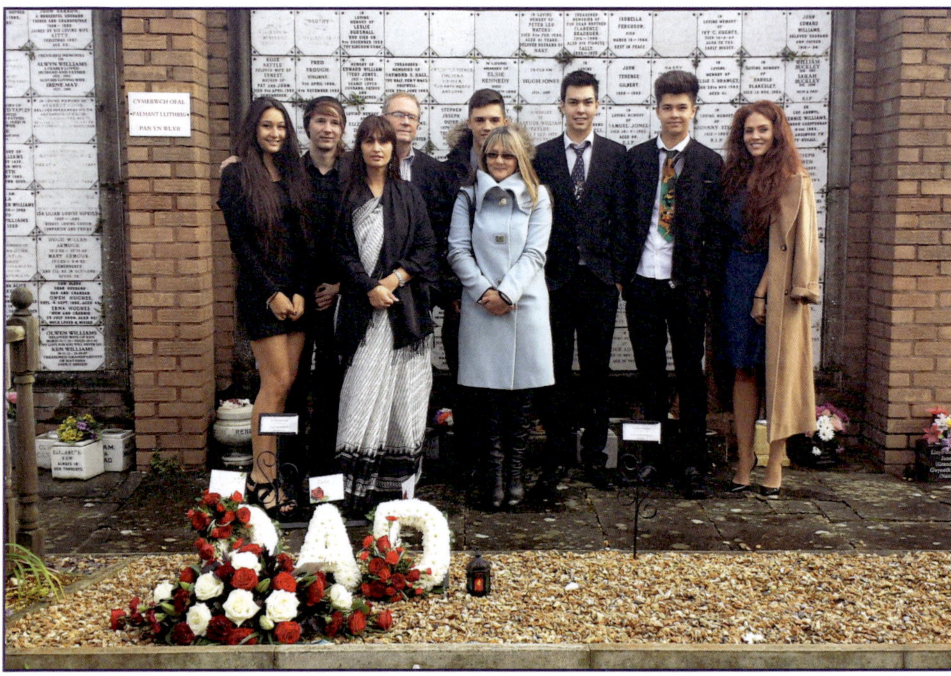
CYMERWCH OFAL

Chapter 15
THE FUNERAL

I had other things still to deal with, like Martin's funeral. Martin and I had discussed the dreaded word 'funeral' but we talked about it in a realistic way too. Initially, Martin wanted just the immediate family – about ten of us – at a private service. Then he thought about it again and reflected on the fact that our children's friends were so sad about what was happening in our life and felt it was only fair to allow them to all attend, so they too could pay their respects and say their farewell. So, we decided to leave it open to all to come.

We used the same funeral directors as we had for Mum. I called them up and organised it all. I had chosen three songs to be played at the funeral which Martin had agreed with. One was called 'Daddy Cool' by Boney M, that was because local people used to say that because Martin helped everyone all the time, he was like the Big Daddy and a very cool dad too. It was fitting with the way most remembered him and his kindness. The second was 'You Are Not Alone' by Michael Jackson. He was one of Martin's favourite singers and he went to one of his live concerts too. The words were so apt. The third song was 'Unforgettable' by Nat King Cole. This was a classic legendary song and so appropriate because whoever met Martin, they could never forget him, and he was a legend in all our eyes.

The other thing was that that all the youngsters wanted to wear a fun tie because they knew Martin had a such a great sense of humour and often wore Bugs Bunny t-shirts and had a lot of cartoon character ties, like Daffy Duck, The Simpsons, etc... They asked if they could wear his ties to his funeral as their tribute and I thought that was so sweet and Martin would love it.

Even my Bollywood girls Cathy, Jennifer, Katharine and Rhiannon wanted to wear their colourful Bollywood dance outfits and bangles to add sparkle. Martin would often try to watch his TV programmes and we would end up rehearsing for our shows and he would say, 'Gosh I am going in the other room. I can't watch my programme with all these veils and dance moves going on around me.'

We would say, 'Oh come on Martin, you love it really; most people pay to watch our performances!' He would smile but carried on doing his own thing. I thought it would be nice to add colour to the day. Our house was full of fun, humour, colour and happy family vibes and I wanted that to be present as we gave Martin a good send off.

Another thing was we told the Minister that if he could announce to everyone that after the service, we as a family needed to take some private time and there would be no such thing as a 'wake' for everyone to meet up and chit chat afterwards. We needed some privacy. Jacky and Steve invited us to be with them at their house afterwards.

Our children wanted to say a few words in the eulogy and to pay their love and respect to their dad in their own words and to stand up and do that themselves, so they planned to do their own write-up. I put together something on my behalf and a little background to Martin's life and asked the Minister to read it for me.

Charlie also wanted to take his little green MGB that his dad had helped him buy as his special tribute to his dad. Mikyle and Charlie wanted to drive behind the hearse in the MGB. Meanwhile Jacky and Steve planned to take Jennah and me in their Mercedes. The grandchildren decided to go in their own cars. All the plans were in place as best as they could be.

On the funeral day, the family came up to the house and I wore a black and white sari, one of Martin's favourite ones. I wore it on our honeymoon in Spain and I knew Martin loved it and also he loved my hair to be loose instead of tied up. I wanted to give him a loving farewell in the way he would have expected to see me. He would have adored me.

Everyone looked smart and we were ready to head down and follow the hearse. We were parked up by the main road leading to the crematorium. I remember thinking and getting anxious as to what my feelings would be when the hearse turned up. So when it did, it was like my heart leapt out of the window, knowing Martin's body was there in the coffin, an awful reminder that he was no longer here. More tears were shed and Steve carried on driving following the hearse which was followed by our sons in Charlie's MGB. We turned up at the crematorium and I noticed our family and friends all waiting and there were lots of them. I didn't feel like engaging in any conversation other than walking into the building. Adam, our eldest grandson, came over and opened my door and escorted me up. There was Martin's coffin with his children, grandchildren and myself and I could hear the song 'Daddy Cool' playing. We followed in behind the coffin and I remember a quiet comment Jennah made to me as we walked up the aisle; it cut me up with great sadness. She said, 'I suppose Mum, this is the closest I'll get to walking up the aisle with my dad, won't it, because he won't be around when I get married.' I really didn't know what to say but my tears said it all. I held her hand to comfort her and took a deep breath as we took our seats.

Then I noticed people walking up the aisle and standing in the sides and alcoves. As I glanced to see why, I realised the room was packed to the brim. It was overflowing with people who came to pay their respects; it was another reminder of how much Martin was loved.

The Minister started the service and talked about Martin's life and his love of classic cars, how much he loved his family and how he was committed to taking care of his mother right to the end. Then it was time for our children to pay tribute to their dad. Jennah got up and spoke lovingly about her dad and she was full of emotion but kept it together until the last sentence when she cried. Then it was Charlie's turn. He talked about his dad being his 'best mate' not just a dad and how he loved the time he spent with him learning how to work with cars. Finally, it was Mikyle's turn. He spoke about appreciating his dad's good lessons he learnt and then looked over at the coffin at the front of the room. He spoke of giving his dad reassuring words that he would take care of his mum and his brother and sister. I was so proud of how well the children did, paying a lovely, heartfelt tribute to their dad in their own words.

As the children sat down, the second song was played: 'You Are Not Alone'. There was not a dry eye in the place; it touched everyone's heart. After a few final words from the Minister, it was time for the curtains to close, and the last song 'Unforgettable' was played as we were all ushered out at the end of the service. We had asked the donations to go to the RSPCA and Pancreatic Cancer UK.
Everybody hugged us outside and then we said our goodbyes and went home to

get our things to head down to Jacky and Steve's house in Cheshire. We stayed there for the night. We talked, we cried and we reflected on some great memories about this very special man in our lives who had left us all and that we would miss him so much.

Harold Martin Swindells
1945 – 2014

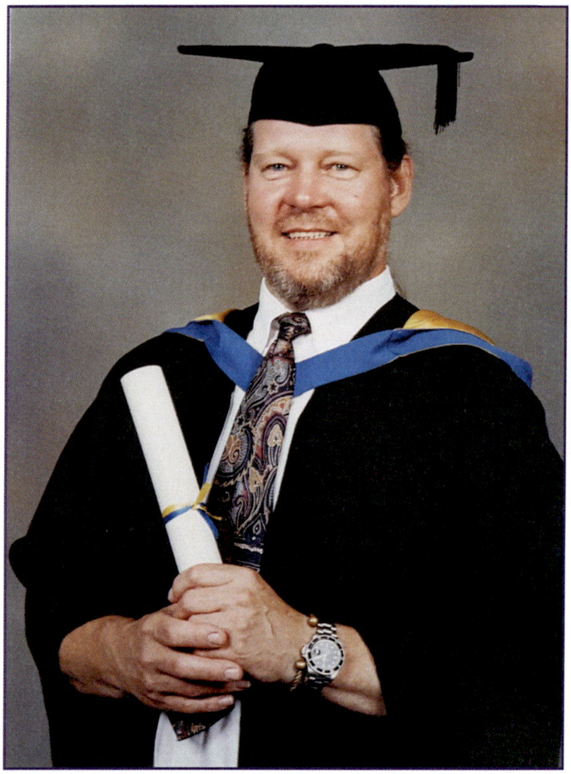

Chapter 16
MOVING FORWARD

Unfortunately, our New Year didn't start off well. I received a call from Mikyle to say *don't worry I am ok*. When they say that, you automatically worry. He was calling from hospital; he had been involved in a car accident and the car was a write-off. I was worried sick but he was ok, just naturally shook up with it all. He was more bothered about the car being written-off, because that was the car his dad had left him and he felt terrible about it. We dealt with the situation as best we could and I tried to relax him out. Mikyle also vowed that he will fix that car and get it back on the road, as a way of showing he wasn't going to let his dad down. He was so determined, he worked day and night and got that car more or less rebuilt, had it MOT'd and back on the road. I felt proud of how he put things right. We were able to move forward from that situation.

I had cooked the New Year's dinner at our own house and sat with the children and said that we must stay focused in moving forward in a strong way and achieve all that we (their dad, nannie and I) had planned to do. I said I would support all they needed with their education and that they must feel comfortable to talk to me any time they wanted to about anything. We shared a lot of love and respect at the thought of moving forward together.

I got a phone call from a very dear friend of mine called Beryl. She had seen me go through a lot of hard work during Mum's and Martin's ill health as well as my own health issues taking a back seat. She helped with my healing with Quantum Touch techniques. I also helped Beryl's business with help on social media training. Naturally we shared lots of conversations and dealt with emotions on what I had been going through. She mentioned to me that she was doing a new course and it was about Positive Intuition and sharing the work of Sonia Choquette, and invited me to the class. She felt that it would be helpful for me on where I was in my life and also that it would be a big help for her to get my feedback on her class too. I didn't think for too long, because I needed a direction to move in. I had started working on my campaign 'Positive Purple' so Positive Intuition fitted in well. It seemed to be a sign. I agreed to attend. I felt that was one of those good gut instincts that worked well for me. I continued my personal development journey with my mentor and facilitator Beryl at these classes and have enjoyed them ever since. I thank Beryl for reaching out to give me that helping hand when I needed it.

My new chapter had begun and I started having to make decisions on things based on my intuition. I started to deal with all the financial affairs with the help of Steve, who had promised Martin that he would take care of us and help us in anything we needed, and he did.

I remember going to the Welfare Office to find out what I was entitled to for help until I got things sorted. Now being a single mum, I needed to understand my financial situation with the children still at school and being a widow. I was shocked when I got told that I was not entitled to the usual help given to single parents because Martin's pension put my income over the threshold for financial help. I couldn't get the usual widow's lump sum either because I was not a pensioner and had two children still in full time education. The only thing I was entitled to was what they called Bereavement Parent Allowance because of the children still in full time education. I asked if I was able to get some help with my mortgage until I was earning a good income. I was told that they couldn't help and that I needed to tell my mortgage company about my situation. This was so difficult because my earnings had taken a big dive whilst I was in the carers' role and I knew it would take some time to get my income up again. This was so sad as we had to close the business that we had worked hard for years and were at a point in our lives where once we were able to buy things with ease and now, I was thinking *what if I lose the house, how will I feed the children and pay for their education?*

I came away feeling lost, sad and helpless. I went home and rang my mortgage company and explained my circumstances to them and they were not that helpful either but made a note on the file to see what they could do.

I thought the only thing I could do was sell Martin's Bentley, which for us had great sentimental value but I knew it would help financially until my income got to be more stable. Unfortunately, in the process of trying to sell the car I came across a guy who tried to help me sell the Bentley but he was very pushy and tried taking over my life – wanting to help with my finances, the kids etc… I felt a great intrusion from him and left feeling vunerable. The more he spoke, the more I realised I did not trust him. He would go on about weird stories of running riot in people's lives and making them squirm. This did not sit well with me and the situation with the car got ugly. In the end, I had to get my family involved to help. It was an absolute nightmare and an upsetting time. We eventually got him out of our lives. I asked Steve and Jacky to step in and help in this difficult matter and between us, we eventually got a written agreement to take the car back from him and paid him what he had spent on it. What a relief that was.

Trip to Malta

One of the things about moving forward was that I had to do a lot of things on my own now. But I am grateful to have been blessed with my bestie Glenys, who I've talked about throughout this book. She is very special and has been such a true, unconditional supportive family friend. In fact, our children adopted her as their 'Godmother'. She has really stood the test of time in our friendship over 19 years. She has seen the children grow up, been a partner in our business, and has shared the good times, sad times and mad times. She has never wanted for anything but pure friendship.

In March 2015, she decided to do something special for me, having seen what a tough time we had been going through. She felt a little holiday was what I needed to get some rest and recharge some of my energy. I remember thinking I had the wheelbarrow race to do yet. She knew I would need something to do to keep me busy so she took it in her own hands to check out the prices. She came back to me to say it was all sorted and she had booked it. I couldn't believe it. I thought, what a kind friend she is and how blessed I am to have her in my life.

Off we went to Malta and I remember feeling strange leaving my kids and going away on holiday without them but knew I needed the break. One morning I woke up crying and sat on the edge of the bed. Glenys came to my side and said, 'Are you ok?'

I said, 'I just had a nightmare and it upset me.' She comforted me and said that it was understandable to feel this way as it was part of the grieving process. She handed me a tissue and I told her about the dream. I was talking to Martin and asking him if I did ok with his funeral. In my dream there were two funerals; one was a cremation and the other a coffin to be buried. How could that have been the case I asked myself? In the dream there was also a coach with my mum-in-law and our children in it. The coach was going round on bends and suddenly it couldn't go any further because of the narrow roads, so it had to pull over to one side and park up. The next thing is I found myself walking through these narrow roads that led to a square like a village square and there was Martin stood there by the lamp post holding his denim jacket over his shoulder looking at me with his usual admiration. Then suddenly I woke up – in tears – because it felt so real. Glenys looked sad as I told her about my dream and hugged me.

A strange thing happened that day. Glenys and I had decided to hire a car and drive around the island. Firstly, we thought we'd head to the city to go to the shops and explore. As I drove us in our little white hire car, we looked at each other because en route there was a church and a funeral taking place. Glenys said, 'Well, that's the dream of your funeral addressed.' We continued into the city and did our shopping and sightseeing. On our way, we came across a diversion and as we followed the diversion, it led us to another church and once again there was a funeral taking place. We literally had to pass the hearse with the coffin in it. Glenys said, 'Well, that's your two funerals from your dream addressed so hopefully we can now relax a bit more on this holiday.'

We got back to the hotel to get changed as we had booked an excursion to see the three cities and a coach was picking us up. When we arrived in Valetta, the coach driver pulled up to the side and said we will be picking you up here as I can't drive any further due to the narrow lanes. I got a shiver run through my body as he said that; it was another reminder of my dream. We got out and as we walked through these little lanes, the tour guide shared some history with us and then we ended up in a little drinking place. As we came out, I looked outside and we were in a cobbled square and sure enough there was a lamp post just like the one in my dream. I couldn't believe my eyes, it was like a deja vu. It was like I had lived my dream from last night all in a day's work. I was emotionally moved by it all. I cannot explain the feeling properly to anyone, but it was truly unbelievable.

There were many things I was juggling to keep things going as smoothly as possible. Looking after my children, their emotions, their important studies and how best to keep them focused to work towards their better futures. Keeping the bills paid in my home, a roof over our head and the upkeep of it all, keeping my work going from marketing/coaching work, to my Bollywood dance and fitness classes etc… I kept asking myself, 'Is this stress ever going to ease up?' I was physically tired out, suffering with my foot from Plantar Fasciitis, fallen arch and a heel spur and this was causing me a great difficulty running my fitness classes and rehearsing the choreographed routines for new materials. In addition, I was driving over to my mum's house (which was about three hours each way) to help her with her disability and her paperwork since my dad passed away. My mum didn't know what to do. Some of my brothers and sister helped with all they could but my mum wanted me to support her and be with her.

With all this going on, the thought of death surrounding me all the time, I knew I had to bravely march on for my children. I realised that as I was feeling ill too, I better do my will and protect my children. So, I sorted that and gave the children the instructions on what to do in the event anything happened to me. I also made arrangements to change my mum-in-law's disabled bathroom into a brand new modern, trendy bathroom for me. My cousin Andrew Stone did all the work and made a fab job of it. I am so grateful for his support too. The admin stuff was starting to come together as well as the house and I started to feel like things were moving on a little bit.

I managed to get away on a business trip to Singapore with one of my business partners, the lovely Emma Louise Dyson. It was a special trip in many ways. The trip was booked before Martin passed away and I was reluctant to go but Martin made me book the trip and said I needed to step out in the big world and explore and 'live my life' without fear and feel totally free. He always wanted me to grow and gain confidence and so it was time to venture out with his blessings. Emma was a fantastic friend to do this with, because she was very travelled and confident so it helped me a lot. She and I had great laughs building our business and a deeper friendship bond. We did a 'Facebook Live' on top of Marina Bay Sands Hotel with a cocktail whilst we worked on our business. Such memorable moments we created. On our way back on the plane, I was telling Emma a little bit more about Martin and I remember we sat there both of us in tears, and Emma said, 'I have never met Martin but I feel I know him so well. What an amazing man!' She was so right. He was an amazing man.

The first wedding anniversary without Martin

This was one of those milestones I was dreading without Martin here. The anniversary of what would have been 26 years together. I wasn't sure how I would cope or what I would do on that day. I decided to spend time with my children and for us all to go away. I decided to book the Double Tree Hilton in Chester where Martin and I had gone to celebrate our Silver Wedding anniversary. I ran the idea by the children and they all agreed that it would be nice for us to spend time there and remember Martin on this date. We had a lovely time and dined at the same restaurant as Martin and I did and talked about Martin, his wit and his wonderful wisdom. The hotel made our stay very comfortable being aware of our circumstances. It was special for all of us to have this time to reflect on how we had moved on and the positive way we had handled things individually. I felt so close to my children and filled with a great deal of pride to see the beautiful grown up adults they had become. They cared for me, were respectful of our situation and supportive to each other. I felt Martin, Mum and I did a great job with our children.

Chapter 17

CHILDREN'S IMPORTANT MILESTONES

Jennah's ROA (Record of Achievement, High School)

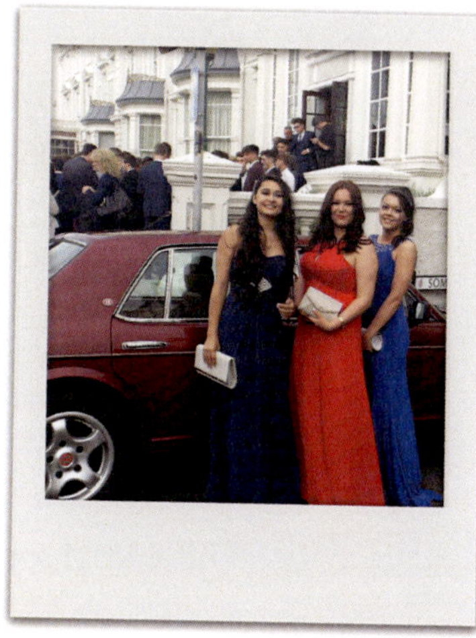

Jennah's end of year ball from secondary school was approaching and I remember being with her when she ordered her gown. She was really looking forward to this event and excited about the beautiful gowns she and all her friends would be wearing for this special occasion.

Naturally, this event was tinted with sadness again because if there was one thing Jennah wanted more than anything was for her dad to have seen her in her beautiful gown and to hear her dad saying, 'You look beautiful my darling.' Words that matter so much for a daughter to hear her father say. She adored her dad because his every word mattered.

She looked beautiful in her navy coloured, long, classy dress. She had her hair in curls by our hairdresser friend Debbie, who did a superb job as always. We took lots of pictures of our grown-up girl who now looked so elegant in her gown.

The nearest thing I could do for her to make her feel the presence of her father was to drive her to the ball in her dad's red Bentley. She looked a million dollars and I personally felt Martin was in the car with us. We picked up her friends and took them all to St George's Hotel where the school pupils gathered for the all-important photographs. Jennah stepped out and went to greet everyone and I knew she was happy at this very special moment. I knew that I couldn't have done more than I did. As I drove off, I said out loud in the car, 'Hey Martin, our girl has made us very proud.' I took a deep breath and drove off home and knew our Jennah would have a lovely ball.

The other thing that is wonderful but sad at the same time was Jennah's moving towards the direction of her chosen career. Her dad always supported her in so many ways for her to head in the direction of being a Vet, because of her love for the animals and wanting to always make them healthier. Well, through her hard work and studies, she was so pleased she got a placement at Liverpool University, which is where she wanted to go to. I remember when she was talking to her dad about the different universities doing Veterinary courses, Edinburgh was mentioned and I turned round and I said, 'We're not moving to Scotland, it's too cold'. Martin and Jennah laughed and jokingly said, 'Who invited you to come to Scotland?' I thought *how cheeky*.

So with all that effort and the planning, it is sad that her dad was not there to see our daughter making it to the University of her choice. I am sure he is watching over her and feeling very proud of her.

Charlie's May Ball (end of sixth form)

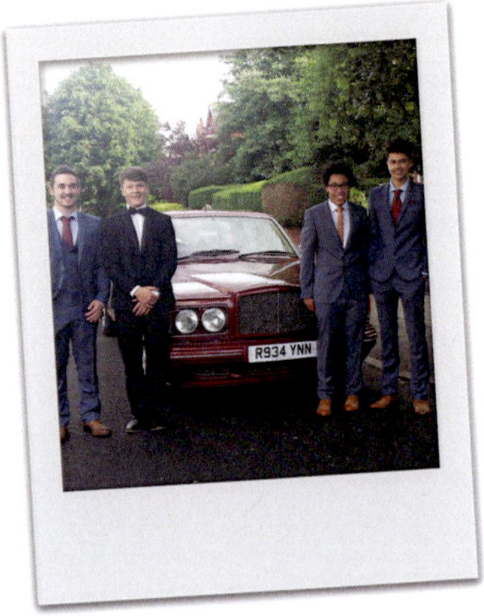

Now it was Charlie's turn for his school leaving do, aka the May Ball. Once again Mum-duty kicked in and we went hunting to get Charlie a really smart suit to wear. He was very clear on what he wanted and he certainly chose well. When he got all dressed up and came down to show me and to ask if I thought he looked ok, well my heart was filled with great pride. I just looked at my 6'3" son who appeared a fine-looking, handsome man. In my head all I could think and say was, 'Oh Martin, doesn't Charlie look very handsome? I hope you are watching down with a smile on your face and pride in your heart.'

Once again I had Martin's red Bentley ready to escort Charlie off to his Ball. We had to pick up his friends en route too and they were all excited at being picked up in Martin's Bentley. The boys all looked very smart. I remember driving the car nice and slowly until one of Charlie's friends Jacob said, 'I thought this car was fast?'

I said, 'Jacob you want fast?' I tapped the throttle and gave the car a little kick in the 400 BHP and gave the kids a little fun, fast treat. The kids laughed and were happy and excited for this fun ride to their event. I am sure Charlie also felt the presence of his dad being around in some way.

I was so glad that the car hadn't sold before these two events for Jennah and Charlie as I know they were moved by having their dad's car there taking them to their special events. They can look back at the pictures with fondness.

However, now the car had to be sold as a matter of urgency. I placed it in the Bentley and Rolls Royce Auction at Burghley House at a Classic Car Show/ Auction. Unfortunately, it didn't sell at the auction due to the uncertainty of the Brexit news. The auctioneer said it was the first time they'd had such a bad result. However, being there was important because we met some people who wanted to help us sell it and it was taken to one of the classic car specialists who eventually helped us. We lost money on it, but I am glad it eventually went to a good home. This sale helped us financially to come through things a bit better. I was able to pay some bills and start sorting things out and it took a lot of stress off me.

There were still other challenges that we all went through but together we continued and I started to get my work moving along too whilst keeping positive in my pursuit to take care of my family and my work.

A similar thing for Charlie, he loved working with his dad and I am sure he would have been proud to see Charlie pull it all together with hard word and dedication in getting to University to study Automotive Engineering because he loved working on the cars with his dad. To study about the automative world was like his dad being with him. Martin often used to say to me 'you know Wifey, Charlie loves tinkering with engines with me, although he is all over the place when using the tools but if he learns to use the tools and an understanding of doing the job properly, he would make a fantastic engineer and I know he loves to show me how well he has done something all by himself'. Charlie loved his dad to praise him with the work; he knew his dad knew how best to do these jobs. He looked up to him with great pride. I am sure again Martin would be proud in the way Charlie is coming along with the love of this work and becoming a fine young gentleman.

One of the lovely things Charlie enjoys as a gift that his dad left him is his MGB. He drives it with such pride and knows that part of his dad is always with him.

Mikyle's Graduation

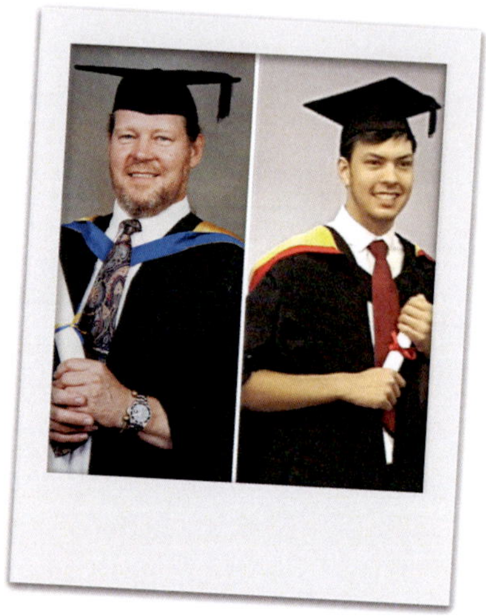

On July 21st 2017 it was a day that we had all waited on for ages. It was our eldest son's graduation from Bangor University. I was so happy and longed to see Mikyle graduate and to see him in his 'Cap and Gown'. These wonderful celebratory moments always missed one most important person and that of course was our Martin. How he would have loved to see his son succeed in his chosen studies with a great future ahead of him and been there at his ceremony. Mikyle also made a promise to his dad and his nannie that he would make them proud and achieve this goal of graduating from university. It was sad that Mikyle's dad helped settle him into the uni, helping take bits for him to his student accommodation but sadly not there to see him finish and to see him complete the journey of his studies in Product Design. I constantly kept motivating Mikyle to focus on getting through the university even with some of the challenges he had after his car accident. I told him to stay focused. He said, 'Mum, I promise I will do my best and have my graduation picture with my cap and gown next to dad's cap and gown picture.' I was so pleased that these words came from him. He looked in my eyes and I knew he meant it.

Well sure enough, he graduated and we all went to his graduation ceremony at Bangor University. Mikyle had also invited Glenys to be there too as she is his Godmother! The day was rainy, but it didn't dampen our spirits in celebrating Mikyle's success. The real tears were that his dad wasn't there to see him. All I know and feel is that his dad would have been looking down at him with great pride and with a big smile on his face saying, 'You did it son, and I am with you and very proud of you.' After the ceremony, we all went for a lovely meal to finish the celebrations and to reflect once again on another great milestone we had achieved together.

I look with great fondness at Mikyle as to how well he has got on with his first job straight after graduation. As a proud product design engineer, Mikyle came home with a beaming smile and then sudden sadness came over him. I asked him if he was ok and he said, 'Mum, I am so proud about my first project at work and guess what?' I said, 'What is it?' He said, 'It's to design a fuse box for a classic Rolls Royce 1930's car.' A car his dad often talked about owning if he could and Mikyle just wished his dad could see what he had been able to design with pride.

I remember him explaining passionately the details of his designs, drawings, details, specifications etc. and he showed me the complete product. He said the owner of the car came to his work place to pick up the part with the actual car outside. He said, 'Oh Mum, imagine if Dad were here, how proud would he have been of me doing that as my first job?' He knew his dad would have been made up with it all, especially as Martin's dad owned a Rolls Royce back in the day and it would've meant a lot to both of them. I said, 'I bet your dad worked that miracle for you to get to do that project!' He looked at me and smiled. He was so happy and yet I could see his eyes filling with tears, wanting his dad to have been there to see it all.

We all agreed, we would give anything to have our Martin back even if it was just for a day. The other interesting thing was he was more than just their dad, he was their best friend too and they all called him Martin not just Dad. We all had such a special bond in each of our own different way with him. He was the most giving, kind, caring man I have ever met. Always wanting to see us happy more than his own wants and needs, hence he was loved by so many.

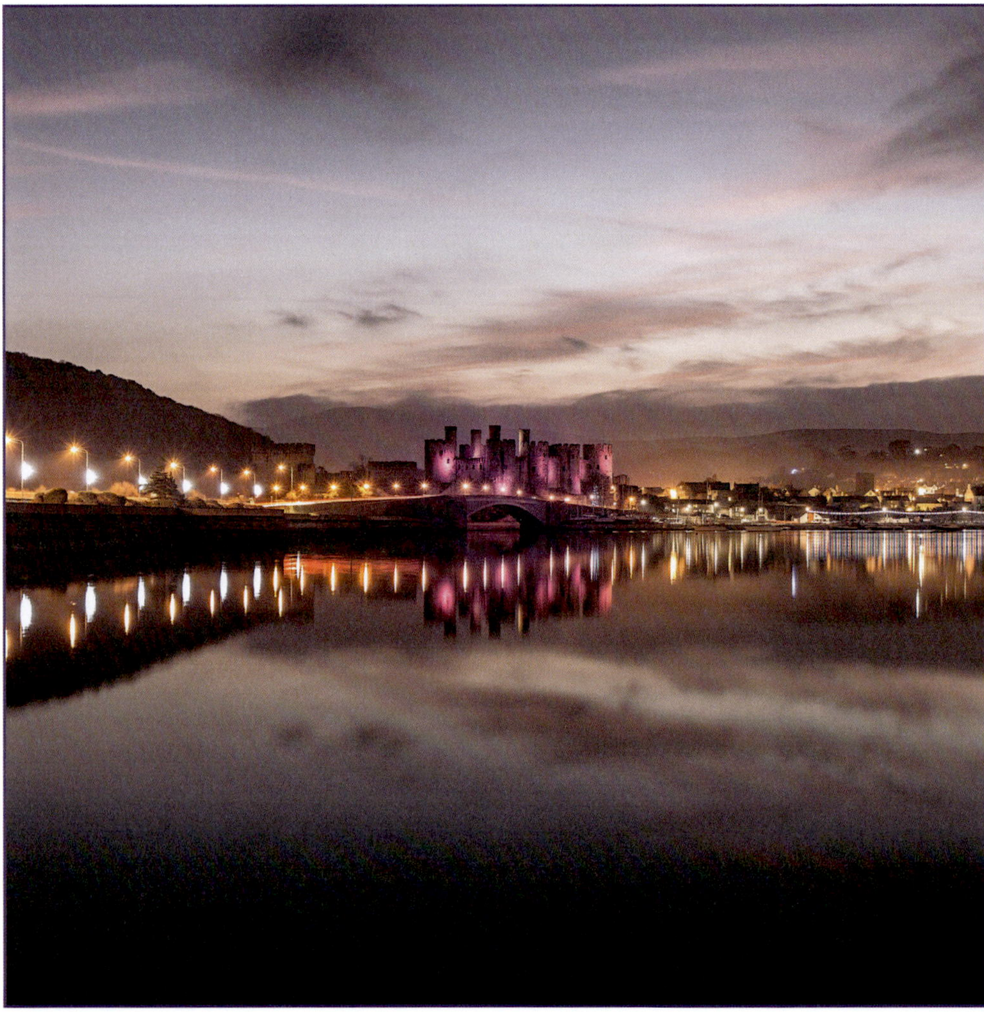

Chapter 18
THE POSITIVE PURPLE CAMPAIGN

A few weeks after the funeral my good friend Jan Read phoned me to say she had been thinking about what was said at Martin's funeral about Martin's wish to raise more awareness for Pancreatic Cancer. She and our other friend Frankie Mullins would like to help me achieve this wish of Martin's. I hadn't even thought that far ahead yet, but Jan said that November is the month of Pancreatic Cancer and we should do it whilst it was fresh for everyone as it would help the message be heard better. She arranged for us to go over to her house and have dinner and discuss a plan. So that is exactly what we did. She also reiterated that she knew how I might not be so strong and still hurting but both she and Frankie would be my strength to help me through it.

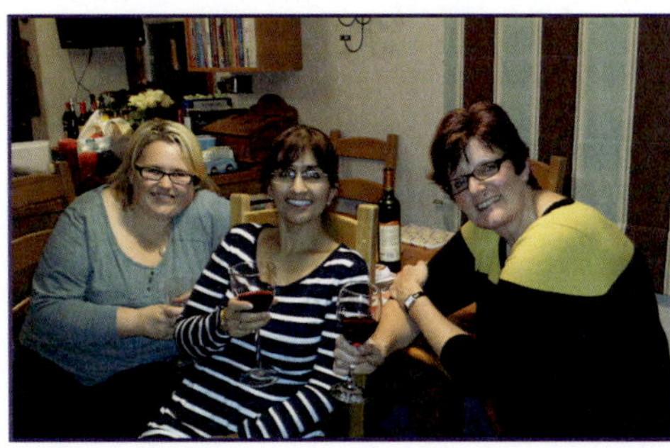

So, we planned our first 'Host for Hope' event. Jan got all the details and with Frankie's help they got us ready to do it. I was so touched and very grateful to these wonderful friends at being so thoughtful in doing this. I want to take this opportunity to thank them for their kindness, understanding and support to help me start the Positive Purple campaign. This was one of Jan's efforts in coming up with the name. We raised a glass to Martin and the Positive Purple campaign was put in place with a date set for 30th November, about a month after Martin passed away.

Purple Lights of Hope - Purple Castle

Whilst all that was being arranged I was looking at the internet and read that it was the 1st World Pancreatic Cancer Day and Niagara Falls in Canada was lit purple! My mind started to work overtime. I thought, what is an iconic building that I could light up purple to make a difference? Then I realised that we have Conwy Castle on my doorstep with water all around it, so why not? Frankie found out who I needed to contact and it was CADW the National Trust. I got hold of the right person eventually after leaving various messages and being transferred to so many different people. When I did finally speak to the right person, I gave them the full story which they were happy to accommodate but said that I hadn't given them much notice. So, I explained that this month was the month to do it and that Martin had only just passed away and it wasn't something I would normally have been thinking of doing so soon after his death, but I needed to capture this important timing. They asked me to email all the information to them and after we cleared all the formalities, I got the go-ahead to turn the castle purple. I got special heat-resistant lighting film that they use in theatres and got the access codes for the castle gates and Jennah came with me to support me on this project.

It took my daughter and I over four and a half hours to get all the flood lights covered with this film. I remember Jennah standing on the wall and saying, 'Hey Mum, there is a lot of water down this side. What if I fall in?'

I turned to her and said, 'Well darling, we helped you learn how to swim and you are a champion swimmer now, so you should be ok if you fall in the water.' She smiled and continued.

Then when we finished, she looked up at the sky and said, 'Hey Dad, hope you appreciate what we are doing and hope this gets the message out there for you.' I smiled at her talking away with her dad. I was so proud of her doing this with me. We were cold, hungry and sad for the reason we were doing it but staying positive for the message of the Positive Purple campaign.

I had arranged for a couple of my friends to take some professional photographs of it, knowing my phone camera wasn't going to do it justice. So asked Justin Van Marle, from Freshpics and Paul Joinson to take these professional pictures for me, which they did kindly.

Welsh Mountain Zoo goes purple

In the process of turning things purple, I decided I would ask the Welsh Mountain Zoo if we could light up the entrance of the zoo too, as this was where Martin's Wheelbarrow and the awareness campaign all started. They also very kindly agreed. Geoff Wiltshire from Tudno TV agreed to take some pictures for us too. Our neighbours and friends came to support us and Mikyle even lit his car headlights purple. We had purple Pancreatic Cancer t-shirts on and I did a little video to say why we were doing this. There was so much support around me and it truly helped me during this time.

Chester Cathedral

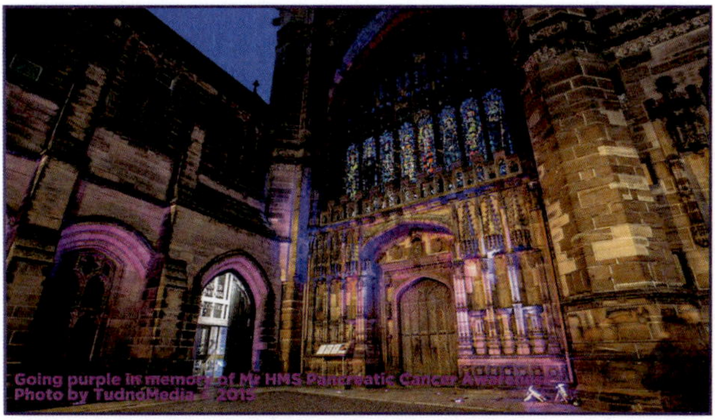
Going purple in memory of Mr HMS Pancreatic Cancer
Photo by TudnoMedia 2015

The other interesting thing that happened was when I went to light up the Chester Cathedral. This came about when, Svitlana from Green Pages talked about wanting to help me run a Host for Hope event in Chester and to help with lighting an iconic building purple as part of the campaign. The Chester Cathedral was chosen to achieve this. I contacted the Cathedral and they very kindly gave me permission to do it. As I was lighting the flood lights with the heat resistence film, I realised there was a little light above the entrance and I couldn't reach it. So, I asked the young lady at the reception if there was a spare ladder that I could use. She said, 'Let me see if any of my colleagues can help.' She put a call out and one of the young men working for the Cathedral came along and she said, 'Gaz, this is Martin and he will help you.' I couldn't believe I was lighting the building in my Martin's memory and along comes a 'Martin' to assist me! It was surreal. He wouldn't let me climb the ladder and said he would put the purple film on the light for me. I felt moved by the kind gesture; it was just like my Martin had come to help me. The event was a success even though it rained so heavy when we were having the pics being done. My dear friend Geoff from Tudno TV very kindly helped me with the photos once again, together with Svitlana Bulava and her husband Usman stayed with me in the rain. Together we got the job done.

Llandudno Pier

I also wanted to light another iconic building/landmark and decided to contact the manager of Llandudno Pier. He said it might be difficult to get the right bulbs, but he would do his best to sort something out. I asked if I could get the colour filters, would he mind? He said he would check with the owner and let me know. The owner of Llandudno Pier agreed to let us go ahead. Again, I had the support of Geoff from Tudno TV as he needed to take some professional pictures for me. It was raining and I had the Host for Hope event to go to in an hour so we rushed over to the Pier and I took all the lighting materials. I climbed up the gates and the Manager was surprised that I was going to those lengths and heights to do this. He phoned the owner and said, 'You've got to come and see this girl who is so dedicated to her campaign. She is literally on top of our gates and lighting the pier purple!' The owner said he was on his way to see the purple sight for himself. The Manager of the pier had got some purple bulbs and did what he had promised, and the pier was lit purple. It was a rainy evening but what made it extra special was the lighting was reflecting beautifully off the wet floor of the pier. The owner eventually arrived and was pleasantly surprised at how lovely his pier was looking in purple. He said, 'Are you Charlie's mum?' I said yes. He then realised the mission because his son was my son's friend. He said he was sorry what had happened to Martin. I appreciated his kindness and support for the campaign and he even said I could light it up anytime I wanted. I invited him to our evening event, but I knew it was short notice. He reached in his pocket and handed me all the money he had at the time which was £100 to be put in the collection box. I was moved by his generosity at this very short notice. It was another great accomplishment. People were so inspired and supportive of my story and commitment to the campaign.

The Wheelbarrow Races

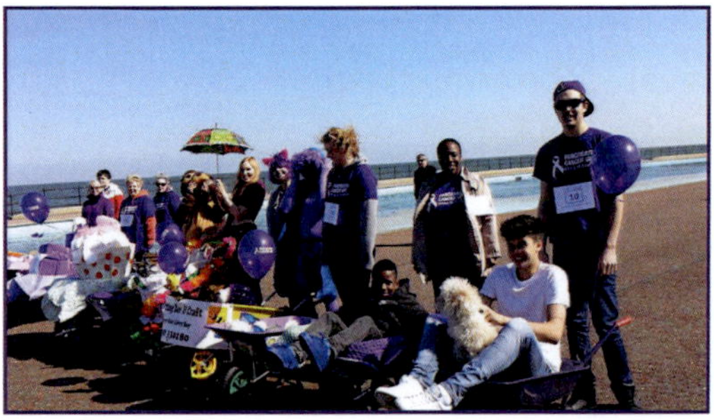

I knew Martin's birthday anniversary was coming up in March and one of the things I wanted to do was mark it with doing a Wheelbarrow Race. I thought it was a fun way to remember him and help raise funds whilst raising awareness. I decided if everyone got a wheelbarrow and raised about £100 sponsorship, if we had 10 wheelbarrows, we could raise £1000. I thought we could add some fun stuff to the race such as: The best-dressed wheelbarrow, the wheelbarrow pusher, and the race winner. Once again, our good friend Geoff Wiltshire from Tudno TV, said he would happily film it for us, and that it would be nice to do a nice promo film for it too. I took Buddy our dog and the wheelbarrow to the place where we wanted to start the race, which was Llandudno Promenade, and we filmed the promo. Buddy had no idea what was happening but he happily joins in with whatever we do with his wagging tail and his little woof woofs.

Our friends did us proud by dressing up in things like Bollywood Beauty with a Brolly and a Trolley (aka Katharine Diane Watson) with sponsorship by Chris Roberts of North Wales Dragons, Honey Bears Tansy Rogerson and her mum, Cupcakes, Garden bugs by Trish Ellison, Superhero and Knitting Bee by Becky Lee and Neil Hughes, Gift of Life by Glenys Griffiths, Subway foods by Elizabeth, Cuddly Toy with Daisies by Beth and Jan, Ruth Smith and Son, Ann Baker, my three children with Buddy etc... The race was monitored and organised by myself and my special friend Cathy Nicol and filmed by Tudno TV. We had the support of our families, and Jacky and Steve supported us once again.

The race went from the paddling pool to the Cenotaph by the pier. The winner of our 1st Race was Katharine Diane Watson as the Bolly Beauty. When everybody made it to the finish line, we got all the balloons and set them off with a Happy Birthday message to Martin. Of course it was all so emotional and I began to cry. Immediately my three children came and hugged me with their love and support. It was a successful event and we were so grateful to all those who supported us in every way.

Race 2

Thanking the following for participants for entering the competition and funds raised for our 2nd Wheelbarrow Race: Svitlana Bulava from Green Pages UK, Jim and Kat in Pyjamas, The naughty Nurse, Fiona Wiltshire as Purple

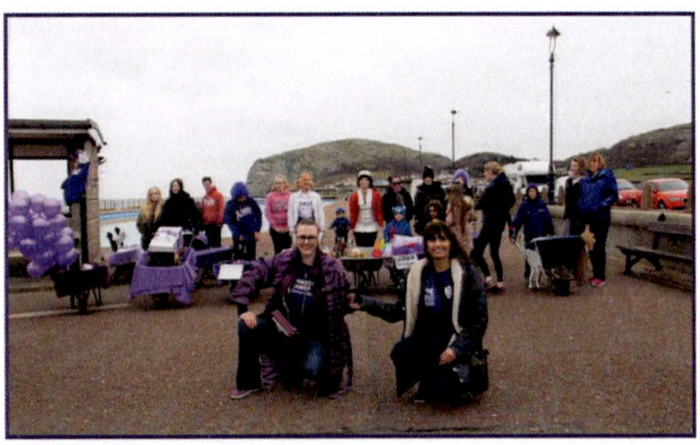

Cheerleader, Glenys with Green plants with Wendi Snowdon from Avon, Bangor University Student and my son Mikyle with Purple balloons, Sunita with her girls Maya and Jaya from Jaya Restaurant, Cara Peppar and her daughter Lexi, Wynn from Hafod by Bryn Kennels and Georgia and her friend James adding Bollywood purple sparkle and jingle. Thanks to all for adding fun to the scene and once again thanks to Geoff from Tudno TV for capturing it on video and taking pictures.

Host for Hope charity events

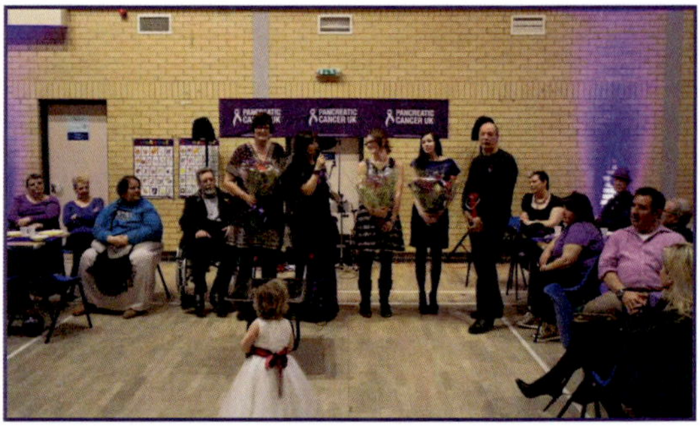

November 30th 2014
Our first 'Host for Hope' was set to take place at our local community centre. We posted some flyers in the area, which Cara Pepper from Lexnia Design and Print did with Mr HMS wheelbarrow logo and all the printing as her contribution to the campaign.

My Bollywood Burnout dancers Cathy, Rhiannon, Katharine, Jennifer and Chloe all decided to put together a little Bollywood interactive dance for the event and for all the tickets sold, it would go to Pancreatic Cancer UK. I agreed to make some curries and rice to help, with a little curry competition too. Another dear friend Teresa Carnall with her Ukulele group decided to dress in purple and help with some entertainment. Many of our other friends joined in to help out for the event. In fact, it was so lovely to see everyone chipping in with their efforts. I was also proud to have my very good friend Geoff from Tudno TV agree to film the event, as Martin was his good friend too. It was Geoff's way of supporting our efforts. Many people gave us gifts for the raffle prizes. The hall was decorated in purple lights with the help of Umbrella Events that Cathy arranged. There were purple balloons everywhere. The event went according to plan and we successfully raised the funds. We also had great support from social media on Twitter thanks to Chris Roberts from North Wales Dragons. He managed to get the awareness reach to over 10 million tweets with likes from Boy George to Nicole Scherzinger and big celebrities.

At the end of the evening I planned to say a few words to thank everyone. I remember how difficult it was for me to talk to everyone, something I don't normally have a problem with doing. But the hurt was still too fresh. However, I managed it ok. I gave flowers, and some wine to all the people that worked behind the scene to help out. I was amazed how it all came together. There was such sadness as it was all so fresh. After the evening, we all came out with the purple balloons and released them in memory of Martin. Geoff took photos and a video that captured all of the event. We thanked all our family and friends for their amazing support to help this first event be a success.

In December, I decided to take a much-needed rest and have some quiet time with the family and that is exactly what we did. We reflected on how the year of 2014 had changed everything in our lives forever. I also had so much legal paperwork to do and change things around from a Mr and Mrs to Ms and there was so much of Martin's stuff that needed attention. Jacky and Steve helped me with this and I am so grateful for their continued support.

We all had our first Christmas without Mum and Martin at Jacky and Steve's with their children (Martin's grandchildren). We raised a glass to them and talked about how we were going to move forward. It would be nice and steady. It seemed so odd not having them with us at the dinner table. Christmas was never going to be the same. We promised that we would maintain a positive posture just as Martin would have expected us to.

One of the nicest gifts given to us was from Jennah's friend Chloe Grogan, who did something very special. She had a star named 'Martin' with all the certification and key rings gifted to us. That was so thoughtful and I know how much she adored Martin. So now when I look up at the sky, I always feel there is a star called Martin shining down on us.

Green Pages and Host for Hope, Chester

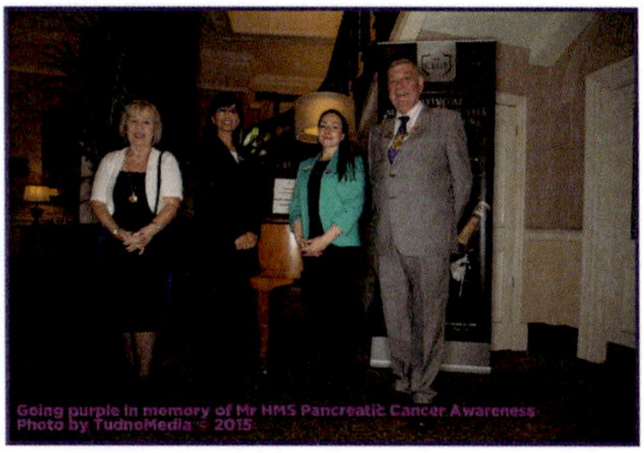

November 2015 - Blossoms

One day I was talking to one of my friends, Svitlana Bulava, the owner of Green Pages UK, and she listened and was very moved with my story. She said she would like to help to support my campaign by hosting a

'Host for Hope' in Chester. We sat and planned to run a networking event at The Blossoms Hotel in Chester on the 17th November with a view to doing the 'Purple Lights of Hope' and light up Chester Cathedral. We had many local business people come and support this event and donated many lovely gifts for the raffle prizes. We also had the honour of the Sheriff of Chester aka Councillor Alex Black supporting us too as our VIP guest. He was very moved by the work I was doing and said, 'I know this girl lights up buildings purple but I didn't know she gets on the buildings herself!'

Soul Night - Llandudno Bay Hotel

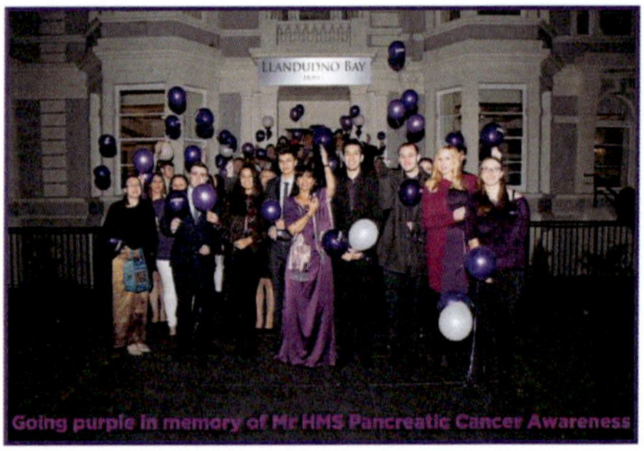

Going purple in memory of Mr HMS Pancreatic Cancer Awareness

I wanted to host our second year of Host for Hope event. This time it was to be held at the Llandudno Bay Hotel. They agreed for us to have the room downstairs to have to ourselves, with a view to them providing food and drinks. I was given the name of a singer by my special friend Ward Roberts from Eagle Enterprise of America, who I used to work with as his Music Marketing Manager. He said one of his friends called Andy Kayne would be a great entertainer for the night. He said the audience love him and he brings every event to life. So, I reached out to Andy and he was delighted to support me. My friend Becky also agreed to step in and sing as she always supports me whenever she can. We had some special VIP guests, our Assembly Member Janet Finch Saunders, another Pancreatic Cancer Patient who did a special oil painting of Martin and James Farrell from Pancreatic Cancer UK.

My Bollywood dancer/friend Cathy helped me in getting the place set up and decorate it with the help once again from Chloe Jackson from Umbrella Events. They provided purple lighting, purple chair covers etc.. Geoff from Tudno TV, filmed the event and we had a Positive Purple photoshoot too. The hotel allowed us to turn all the lighting at the front of the building purple; it looked beautiful. Our family and friends came to support us and at the end of the evening we all went outside to release the purple balloons in the air for another successful event of raising awareness and funds for Pancreatic Cancer UK.

November 2016 - Crowne Plaza

Svitlana felt that she would like to do more for the Host for Hope event this time. She wanted to incorporate it into her Green Pages Gala Awards Night and so set out to get the job planned. We contacted the Crowne Plaza, Chester and they were very delighted to host this event. The event planning was done with our wonderful friends Sue Miller and Lindsay Burgess. Lindsay was our MC for the evening. These special ladies were amazing in the way they helped us run the show smoothly. The awards and nominations got well underway. My Bollywood Burnout dancers, Kat, Cathy, Jennifer and Rhiannon started to prepare for their dances and they delivered a beautiful show. I was so proud of them especially as they danced without me leading them and Kat took the lead for the first time too.

The gifts for the prize draw started coming forward. Svitlana had asked The Mayor of Chester to be our VIP guest for the night and we also had a Special VIP Guest singer – Classical Cross-over Tom Spence who was thrilled to support this special event. We also had an official Pancreatic Cancer UK representative the lovely Debbie Wells, who gave updated information on the treatments and research to help improve on the necessary work to help more patients going through this tough time. Once again, our loyal film crew was there from Tudno TV. I had all my family and friends there and even some of my friends turned up from London, the Midlands and elsewhere.

Local businesses were up for awards too. So many amazing people were nominated for business awards and delighted with their recognition as I was too. I was nominated for the Networking Person of the Year Award and delighted to have won it. The evening was a success and great funds were raised and we captured many special moments. Our friend Debbie Thomas from Grangewood Copywriting wrote a lovely article about the success of the event in the Chester Chronicle.

The day after the event I sailed out on the Queen Mary 2 to New York with my friend and client Eileen Morgan along with my bestie Glenys. Eileen's son was performing at the shows on the cruiseliner and I had a golden opportunity to join her. I knew it was a welcome break for us after the event. It was a fabulous holiday and the first time for me on the Queen Mary 2 and to New York. We all thoroughly made the most of the rest, relaxation and rejuvenation.

Rydal Penrhos Choir

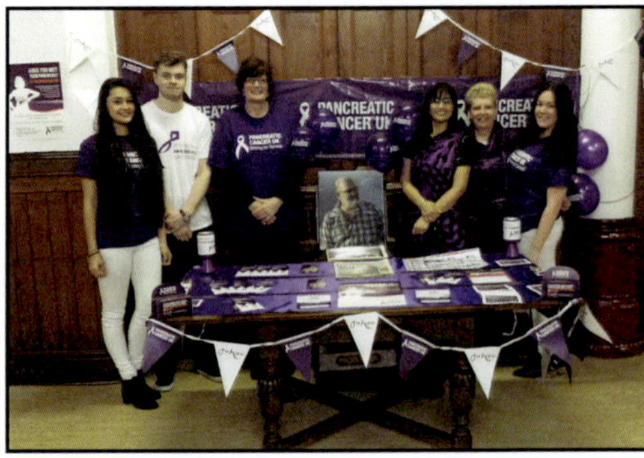

One of my ex-neighbours and a very good friend Sarah Watkins talked about an idea she had. She said, 'I am part of the Rydal Penrhos Choir and every year we try and help raise funds for various charities and good causes. I know you have been campaigning for Pancreatic Cancer awareness at Martin's request and I want to help you.' I was touched by Sarah offering to help out and said that would be lovely. She said Martin was their friend too and it would be a pleasure. So, on that note we started to plan the event which took place at St Joseph's Church, Colwyn Bay. We set out our stall, with the help of Jan Read, Glenys, Jamie, Jennah and Chloe Grogan (one of Jennah's school friends). We had the literature from Pancreatic Cancer UK and collection boxes. We had a few people that put some money in the box (about £20) but most of the people took a leaflet and talked to us about the purpose of our stall. The choir sang beautifully and the Headmaster of Rydal said a few words and invited me up to tell a bit about my story and about the charity. I shared some information and kept my composure whilst I explained how I lost the love of my life to this cruel cancer and how we needed to be more aware of it. The choir finished on some beautiful singing. I went back out to the stall and I couldn't believe how many people had started to put money in the charity box once they understood about it more. In fact, we were delighted to have not only raised awareness of the cancer but over £800 on the night! I am grateful for my friend Sarah Watkins for reaching out to me in helping this success be achieved.

Man of the Match Trophy - North Wales Dragons

Another special thing that happened during my campaign for Martin was from the wonderful work of the North Wales Dragons especially our dear friend Chris Roberts, together with his sons Steve and Gaz. Chris phoned me and said that they wanted to do something special in memory of Martin. The usual 'Man of the Match' trophy that they normally presented, would now be called the 'Martin Swindells Trophy' to pay respect and acknowledge the strength Martin had to fight to win, just like a special player is recognised for going out to win for the team. This really touched my heart and brought tears to my eyes. It was a wonderful thing to do to recognise Martin in this wonderful way. They asked me to present the trophy to the player, and I was proud to accept that duty.

The second year (2017) I was working away and it was represented by Nick from the Welsh Hearts Charity as they were sponsors of the match too.

This year (2018) 3rd year on I was privileged to have been asked again. I gladly went and watched the match and then presented it to the young player recognised as going the extra mile to play hard and help the team to succeed. As I went to present the trophy, I said a few words about its significance and Martin's fight with cancer and that I was proud to be representing him. As the player accepted the Trophy from me, he quietly said, 'You are Charlie's mum aren't you?' I said yes. He smiled at me as he knew our story and I could tell he was moved by it all too and the specialness of the trophy.

It's things like this that reflect strength, respect and courage to fight on like brave soldiers. I am very grateful to Chris Roberts.

Pier to Pier walk x3

Another campaign for raising awareness was the Pier to Pier walk, which was organised by our good friends Chris Roberts and family from the North Wales Dragons. I had a t-shirt printed with Mr HMS and Pancreatic Cancer awareness together with the North Wales Dragons logo on it. I asked for nominations from people as I set myself to do this walk. I was supported by my trusty bestie Glenys. We wore our Purple t-shirts and made our way down to the Pier, walking through the woods, doing a Facebook Live. When we got there, everybody was getting ready to walk.

This event was about everybody being welcome to do the walk and represent their own chosen charity. There were lots of charities represented. Chris also asked me if I would do a Bollywood Dance as a warm up. I was pleased to get everyone warmed up for the walk and everyone enjoyed the funky, interesting moves. Off we went walking. I noticed that with all my fitness levels, my bestie Glenys was overtaking me and on a mission to get to the finish line. I couldn't see her for dust; there she was one minute and then she was crossing the line the next! I was very proud of her and her dedication to do this walk for Martin.

The second year we did the same thing and once again I warmed up everyone with the Bollywood moves by popular request. I often helped Chris Roberts on his events. He is a good man and has always done brilliantly for community projects with his work with the North Wales Dragons.

On the third Pier to Pier walk, I was running late from a prior event, so one of my Bollywood girls Kat, stepped in at the last minute and warmed up everyone. Glenys and I eventually joined in and continued the walk. I am pleased to have been on every walk supporting Chris and raising awareness for Pancreatic Cancer UK.

The Positive Purple Campaign continues

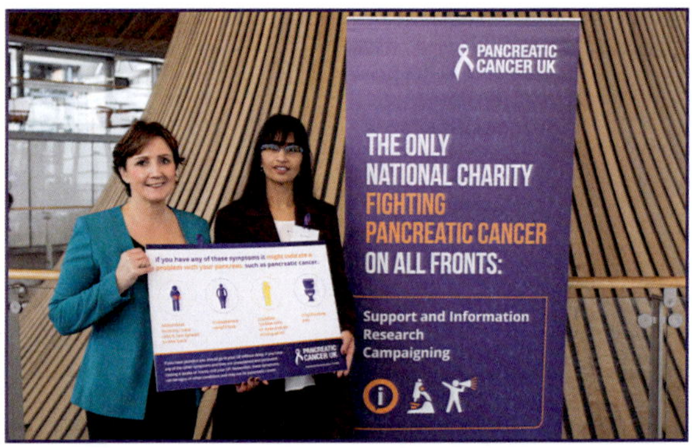
PANCREATIC CANCER UK
THE ONLY NATIONAL CHARITY FIGHTING PANCREATIC CANCER ON ALL FRONTS:
Support and Information
Research
Campaigning

My work with Pancreatic Cancer was also starting to get noticed. I was invited to attend as a guest by Pancreatic Cancer UK (PCUK) at the Welsh Assembly to see the current plans and the work that is being carried out to treat this cancer and how the funds are being used. I was also asked by PCUK (prior to this event) if they could publish Martin's story to present for the Welsh Manifesto. After all, it was after Martin's wish to raise awareness. On my six hour journey to Cardiff, I was accompanied by my dear friend and neighbour Lexcie, and what a lovely relaxing journey we had through the hills, valleys and lakes of beautiful Wales. When we got there, my local Assembly Members Janet Finch Saunders and Darren Millar acknowledged me and offered their support in any way they could to get treatments, awareness and information for the people of Wales. PCUK's head office team were all so delighted to actually meet me, as I was to meet them! We had many pictures taken and shared it on social media especially on Twitter. It was a very proactive effort on everyone's part. I also got to meet my 'Purple Sister' Linda Reardon from South Wales who has been doing amazing work on the purple campaigns from Lights of Hope, to community projects. She is incredible and has been my inspiration and support for doing my work. We are two 'Purple Sisters' in action from North Wales to South Wales.

I also realised that my fundraising page was getting close to the £7,000 and I said if I got to my target of £10,000 I would climb Mount Snowdon and put a flag up to mark the occasion.

Business From Home European Congress - Amsterdam, May 2018

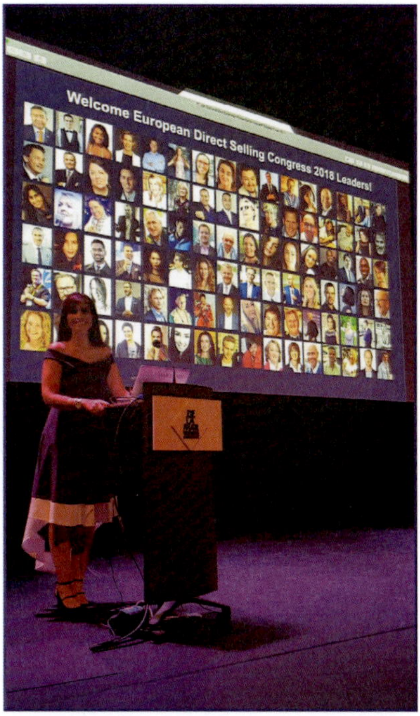

One of my highlights and one of the three goals I wanted to achieve was success with my public speaking duties.

Whilst I was at one of our company's annual conventions in Las Vegas, I got talking to the Owners of Business for Home Ted Nugent and his partner Dini Noorlander. I got talking to them about my life with Martin and the cultural challenges I faced growing up and my Bollywood Burnout business. I even showed Dini some Bollywood dance moves. I was invited by them to attend the 1st European Congress in Amsterdam. I would be an international female speaker from the UK. I was delighted to accept this wonderful invitation. I went through some details with Ted as to the content of delivery and details of the event. I then set to work to present a valuable presentation on my background covering 'suppression to expression', my elopement, my life with Martin, his cancer and my commitment to my work as a leader. I included the success of my work in Direct Sales within my own company to the Network Marketing industry. Just after Christmas, I noticed I was also featured in the Hall of Fame 2018 for Business for Home amongst many industry legends and inspirational leaders and speakers, like Jim Rohn, Bob Proctor, Les Brown, Tony Robbins, Eric Worre etc... I felt privileged to be within that line up.

One of Martin's personal projects was to help me gain confidence to be able to speak anywhere about anything and deliver a confident talk. He used to say: *you are more than capable Wifey, and can hold your own with anyone, anywhere.* He was my biggest cheerleader. When I went to do my talk I remembered all of Martin's words about owning my own space and to speak from my heart. That is exactly what I did. My good friend Becky aka Rebecca Lee agreed to come and support me. Becky became my stand-in PA and supported me throughout the weekend. We even had a little celebratory day for my birthday and went on a lovely cruise on the canal. Becky recorded the event for me. We had such fun! I appreciated a great time with her.

The stage lighting had purple in it and I felt Martin was right there by my side watching over me. I could feel how proud he would be and that he predicted I would be talking on many stages, confident and in command of the audience's attention with ease. I shared my heartfelt story at the congress and people were very moved. I had so many people stop me in the breaks and tell me how inspired they were from my talk. The women especially said it gave them a great feeling to hear my story and I encouraged them to do more about sharing theirs too. To be told that I was a great role model was so nice to hear, as I had always wanted to be that from a young age. I even got the audience to do a few Bollywood moves and took a selfie to add some fun to it.

At the end, I was recognised and awarded as an Ambassador for the Direct Selling and Network Marketing industry. I am very grateful to Ted and Dini in giving me this wonderful opportunity. If they only knew how much it meant to me and the long-term wish it accomplished. It was also such a special opportunity for me to share the efforts of Martin's awareness wish at this fabulous event which was held at the Del La Mar Theatre in Amsterdam.

Full Tough Mudder - East Midlands, May 2018

I was talking to the children about how I needed to hit my £10,000 as I was £3,000 short of my fundraising target. I said that if I hit my target, I would climb the highest mountain in England and Wales – Mount Snowdon – and put a flag up there to say we did it!

Then one day I had a message from Jennah saying, 'Mum can we have Sunday dinner on Monday?' I found that very funny but agreed with her and said, 'Sure, why not?' So on Monday we finished dinner and Jamie asked me to sit down because they wanted to tell me something. I got anxious wondering what they were going to tell me. They said they had been thinking about what I am trying to achieve with my Positive Purple campaign and they knew that I was worried about how I was going to achieve it. Jamie said, 'You know you were worried about the extra £3,000 to hit your target, well you don't need to worry about it anymore, because we have sorted it.' I couldn't understand what he meant until he explained that he had called Pancreatic Cancer UK and asked for a fundraising info pack because he had decided on doing a Tough Mudder obstacle course with Mikyle, Charlie and their friends. They all agreed to do this and got commitment from everyone to raise the difference needed. I couldn't believe what I was hearing! I was emotionally moved and this was music to ears. I was truly made up with this news and felt very proud of Jamie for organising this.

The Full Tough Mudder was carried out by Jamie Joinson, Mikyle Swindells, Bryn Jones, Josh Roberts, Oliver Thomas, Sam Davies and Tim Fisher. Unfortunately, Charlie was not able to do this due to a football injury with him ending up in hospital a few days before. He was gutted to not be able to participate in it. The event took place whilst I was away on business in Amsterdam and all I was wishing was that I was there with the boys watching them come through the finish line. However, I was also raising the awareness through my public speaking at a global event. We were all in action with the campaign in our own ways. Jamie, Mikyle and the boys had a tough but fun time with the 10-mile obstacle course in the mud and achieved recognition with their t-shirts and acknowledgement from Pancreatic Cancer UK and myself giving them a shout out! They succeeded in their mission and I was so proud of them for doing this. We were closer to our target.

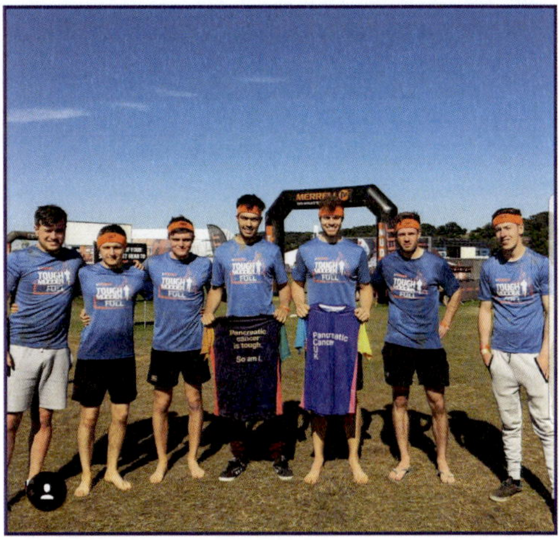

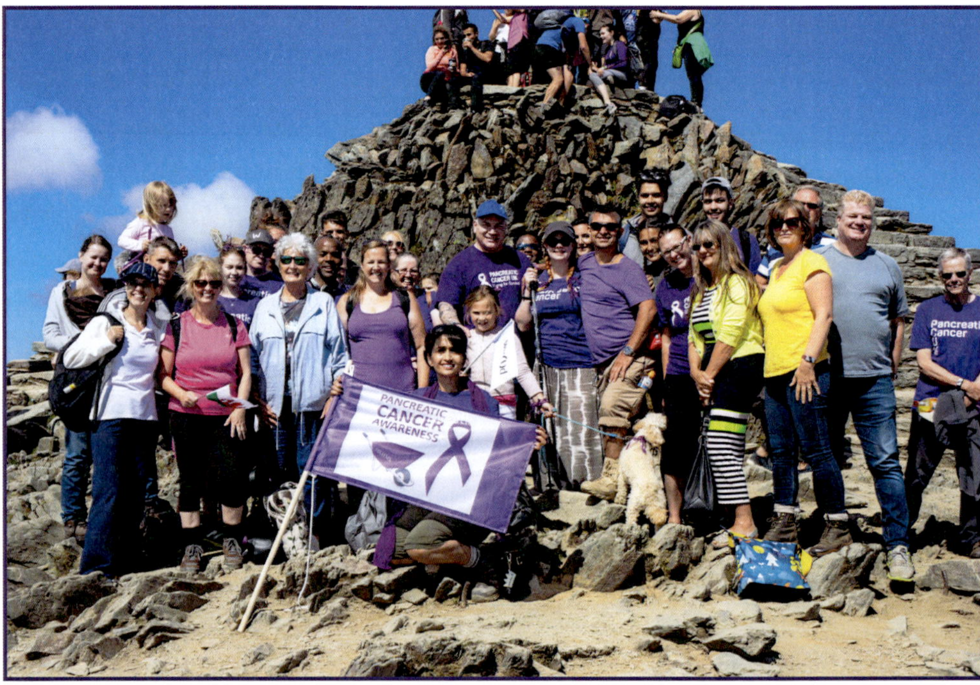
PANCREATIC
CANCER
AWARENESS
Pancreatic
Cancer

Chapter 19

PROJECT 77 - MOUNT SNOWDON

The second major goal of mine was to climb Mount Snowdon if I reached my fundraising goal of £10,000. I wanted to go the extra mile too. I called this mission 'Project 77' for the following reasons: I wanted to put 7 flags with 7 global messages and all this was to take place in the 7th month. I started to get the word out there and checked with my insurance company to cover the insurance, risk assessment etc. I contacted Snowdon Trust to check how to go about doing this event properly and I contacted the Snowdon Railway company to give them details of the numbers of people that would be using the train. I notified people through my 'Facebook Lives' and created an event page. Glenys and I went a few months earlier, to do a recording to show the people where it was and what our plans were. We checked on what type of clothing and footgear we needed to have in place and what to carry up the mountain too.

On the day, we all met at the station. One of my friends Dave Ashford wanted to be involved in some way to help as he lost his partner to Pancreatic Cancer too. Dave helped to get everyone registered that were going to travel on the train. Geoff Tudno agreed to kindly record the event and get one of his crew to take professional pictures. We had about 50 people ready and committed to do this. I had my Ucan2 Global business partners Dave Ives, Peter Webb, Grahame J Brown and Jason Regan join us as they knew what a big deal this was for me and I wanted all those people to be right by my side.

All my family, my bestie and special friends were all set to trek up the mountain with me. The Mayor of Colwyn Bay Steve Williams came to give us a send-off as he couldn't climb up the mountain due to a back injury. Martin's grandson James agreed to do some family filming for us as we walked up the mountain. I also had a friend Lyn whose father was actually fighting pancreatic cancer at the time and she wanted to do the walk for Martin and for her father. Cathy my Bollywood friend had her husband do the walk with us and she came on the train with her two daughters. Glenys had a mini tuck shop in her rucksack so Simon, Cathy's husband, helped Glenys along the journey by carrying her bag and helping her. He was her knight in shining armour. Jason, one of my business partners, carried the first aid box and helped those that had blisters. My three children walked although Jennah and Charlie with Jamie walked up too fast! But Mikyle kept a close eye on me. Grahame J Brown's daughter Steph held my hand on part of this journey and we encouraged each other up the mountain.

It was a glorious sunny day. There were so many mini stories along the journey to the top, such memorable moments captured en route. We huffed and puffed as we bravely marched up with much laughter and lots of pictures taken of special moments. It was wonderful and a heart-warming feeling to have all those amazing people supporting me in this incredible way. Even my friends Fitz and Zoe travelled from Plymouth and my friend Guarang from Northampton came up to do the trek with us...they had me chuckling all the way to the top. Another friend of my friend Paula travelled from Cardiff and lots of others locally, regionally and nationally made the effort to be with us. We had the positive purple in t-shirts and balloons making their way to the top.

The 7 flags with 7 messages were as follows:

Flag 1 - Pakistani Flag. This was to represent where I originate from – Sharing the message: Don't forget your roots. Be proud of your origin.

Flag 2 - Indian Flag. This is because I am known as one of my titles as 'Ghazala Jabeen the Bollywood Queen'. As in the Bollywood movie scene with my work in sharing eastern culture with the western world. (These two flags together also represented the unity of the two countries that once fought one another, now sharing the two being embraced on western soil.)

Flag 3 - Union Jack. This represented the United Kingdom where my father brought us to. To give us a better education and a better lifestyle showing how grateful we must be for our opportunities.

Flag4 - Welsh Flag. This had to be represented, one because two of my children are Welsh, and because we lived and built our business in Wales with the support from the Welsh Assembly. Also, we were standing on the highest mountain in Wales.

Flag 5 - World Changer Flag. This was to represent that in Business I have not only supported people on my doorstep but on an international basis. Living local, working global.

Flag 6 - Lady Leader. This was to represent all the women in the world, from sisterhood, motherhood and every hood that a woman has worn to take care of business and family.

Flag 7 - Mr HMS & Pancreatic Cancer UK Flag. This was the most important flag, representing Martin's wish in raising awareness and Pancreatic Cancer UK funds to help with better research and treatment.

I am pleased to say not only did we achieve the £10,000 fundraising goal but actually exceeded it, achieving £11,000. With great pride and excitement I stood at the top with my flags and all my family and friends from near and far supporting this important project.

I actually stood up there and did a high five to Martin to say WE DID IT!!! I was moved to tears and sat on a little rock and cried... realising that we had actually done it and reflected on coming this far. I did this with a broken heart but feeling very grateful to all those that helped me along the way.

Together we made a mark. We made a difference!

I couldn't have done all this without the behind the scenes support and help of Glenys, my Bestie, being by my side all the way and helping make this event a success.

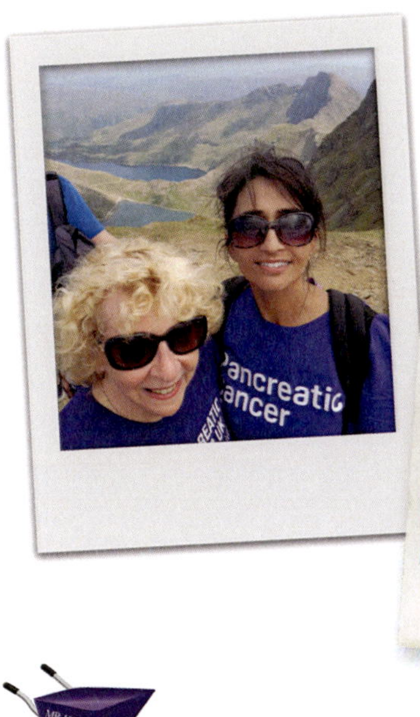

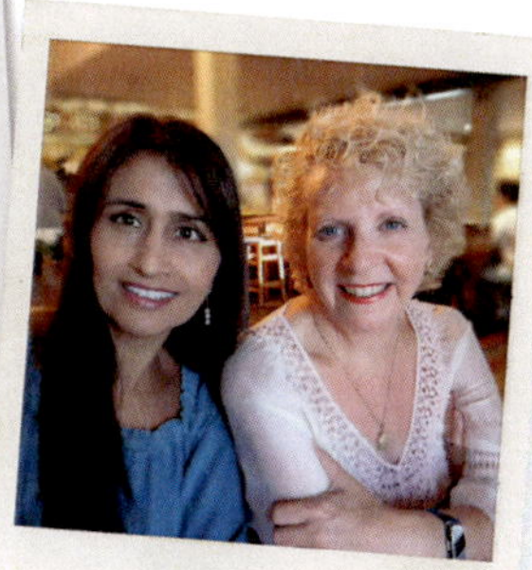

Besties

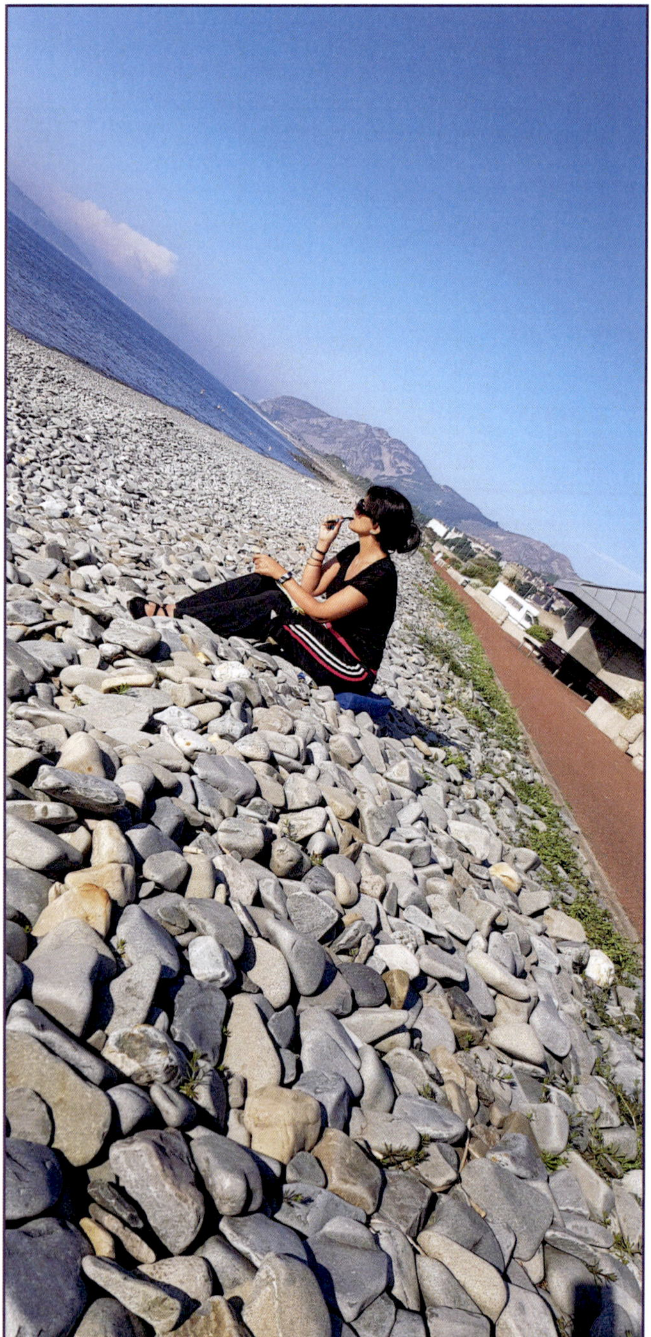

Chapter 20
REFLECTIONS

As I sit at my desk finishing the last chapter of this book, floods of thoughts come to my mind. I reflect on the emotions that I have been through to pull everything together. It has been a 'stop/start' experience with plenty of tears throughout the process. I have to say this has been the hardest write-up I have done in all my life.

It was only a few months back when I was sitting on the pebbles by the seashore in Penmaenmawr, North Wales with a pen to paper scribbling away the contents of this book. This was the third thing of the three main things for this year's goals. There were more tears than ink on the paper and every now and then, when it became too much, I would look up at the sea and watch the waves come and go, children playing on the beach, dogs chasing the ball, couples holding hands...as I took a breather. Glenys, my best friend knew how difficult this was for me and one day she did something very special. Firstly she motivated me through this process to get writing when I was procrastinating. One day I got into a good flow of writing and didn't want to take a break for lunch and then suddenly she turned up with some fish, chips and coffee to help keep me going. I was very touched with this kind gesture by my friend, as she had driven a 2-hour round trip to bring me some food to save me losing any time. I will always be thankful for her kindness throughout our friendship, especially at challenging times; she always eases things for me.

I've reflected on what a lovely life Martin and I led for over 25 years. I couldn't have been more loved than I was by Martin. We brought three beautiful children to this world who have made us very proud, especially as they have become very capable young adults leading their own lives independently. There is a sense of a 'job well done' and yet some sadness that Martin isn't here to see them all grown up doing their own amazing things.

I remember saying to Martin, 'How will I cope on my own when you are gone and it gets dark and lonely?' And his reply, 'You will never be in a dark, lonely place Wifey, because you are the shining light for others and that light will reflect back on you. You will be surrounded by lots of people all the time.' He wasn't wrong at all, as I look at the buildings I have lit and all the people that have been with me supporting the Positive Purple campaign I realise there is lots of light and people around me all the time.

Writing this book has allowed me to deal with my grief which I was avoiding by being busy. It has been like holding back the dam whilst I see my children get to safety before letting my tears go.

I feel proud on how positively we have worked together in order to move on and how much has been achieved in our campaign, our personal life, business life and the support for our children in helping them stay focused with their education and future careers. It's just as Martin and I had wished for to give them the best start in life.

I realised there has been a lot of ground covered with our Positive Purple campaign over the 4 years since Martin passed away, but he would be so proud of this achievement. I feel emotional as I pay my tribute to my Martin in this book and as I prepare to move forward knowing that Martin will always be watching over us as our Guardian Angel making sure there is always light in our life. He will be always be forever in our hearts.

Finally, I want to show my appreciation to everyone that has been with us and given us the strength to march on like brave soldiers, for the support in our fundraising campaigns the donations received and the continued care shown to us.

Much love, light and respect.

Ghazala Jabeen

MR H.M.S
– AKA HAROLD MARTIN SWINDELLS

H. Martin Swindells, aka Mr H.M.S, was known mostly as Martin 'the big man with a big heart'.

Martin was born in Stockport in Cheshire, UK. Martin had a great love for classic cars from being a young child working alongside his dad, who owned a Rolls Royce and a couple of classic kit cars with an interest in steam engines and supercars. He loved the engineering, mechanics and the beauty of these vehicles. He was also a Company Director of a national haulage company, responsible for a fleet of over 400 vehicles.

Martin and Ghazala eloped and had been married for over 25 years. He adored his wife and their three children, Mikyle, Charlie and Jennah. Martin's eldest daughter Jacky (from his 1st marriage) has been a very special person in his life and he always turned to her for advice. Martin's world was his family and his pets.

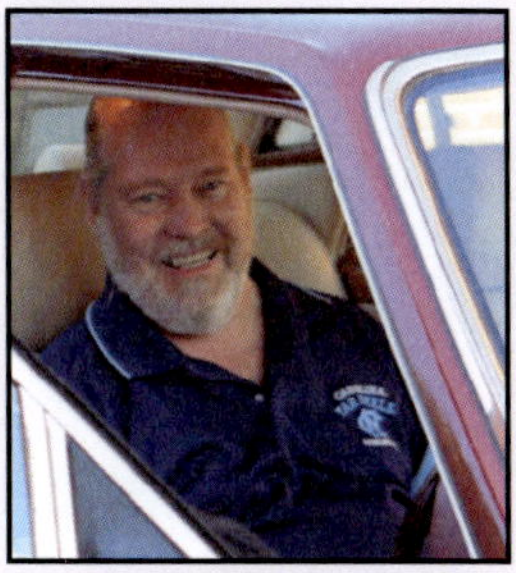

To sum up this incredible man, he was gentle but assertive, kind but careful, intelligent but quiet, giving but not taking. Most of all he was a very loving man who would help anyone anytime. He was loved and respected by all.

ACKNOWLEDGEMENTS

I am delighted to acknowledge my appreciation and thanks to everybody that helped with the launch of this special book and the success of the Positive Purple Campaign.

This mission wouldn't have been so successful and accomplished in this beautiful way without the following people and businesses who helped make it happen:

Team Author UK – Sue Miller for all the editing, proofreading, design and management required to help me publish my book. The radio interview on Calon FM and for helping with our Chester Host for Hope event. Also to Carole Chevalier of TAUK for the gorgeous design and layout of this book.
www.teamauthoruk.co.uk

Mikyle Swindells BSc – Huge love and thanks to my son who is a Freelance Designer specialising in both Product Engineering and Graphic Design for designing this amazing book cover.
www.mikyle.co.uk

Pancreatic Cancer UK – For all the support for our fundraising and media support.
www.pancreaticcancer.org.uk

Andrew Stone – Our cousin from Andrew Stone Photography for all the memorable photos captured for Martin's Wheelbarrow Challenge and for Family Memory pics as well as the photo of Martin sitting in his red Bentley on the back cover.

Andy Kayne – Our Soul Singer friend, Andy did a fantastic singing tribute to Martin and us all.

Brad Burton – Who gave me sound advice regarding writing a book and support as and when I have needed it.
www.bradburton.biz

Cathy Whitfield – Cathy my Bollywood friend/dancer helped set up these events and followed her commitment to Martin, that she would always be there for me and support me.

Chester Cathedral – For going purple.
www.chestercathedral.com

Chris Roberts – The North Wales Dragons for all his support in so many ways.

Conwy Castle – For permission to light the castle purple.
www.cadw.gov.wales/daysout/conwycastle

David Ledward – North Wales Tweets helped with all the social media support for all our campaigns as well attending in person.

Debbie Thomas, Grangewood Copywriting – For my website profile and the writeup in the Chester Chronicle.
www.grangewoodcopywriting.co.uk

Double Tree by Hilton, Chester – For making our 25th Silver Wedding Anniversary be so special and for the added extra touches to our experience.

Geoff, Tudno TV – Videographer for all the videos and photographs at many of the different events.
www.tudnotv.com

Glenys Griffiths – 'My Bestie' – Glenys my best friend never left my side whenever I needed her. She gave me her listening ears, her shoulders to cry on and love to help me feel comforted.

Jacky, Steve, Adam, Stephanie, James – My family have supported us throughout the process and shown great care and love during these difficult times.

James Barnes – Filming of Project 77 and the message for the book launch.
www.james-barnes.co.uk

Jamie Joinson – For the family support to Jennah and us all throughout the process and organising the Full Tough Mudder to help us get to our fundraising target.

Jannie Rawlinson – Calon FM Classical sounds for you. Radio Interview.
www.calonfm.com

Jennifer, Katharine, Rhiannon – My Bollywood dancers who supported the events from dancing, fundraising and general support to me and my family. They helped keep my spirits lifted.

John Evans, Handy Office – For his printing support for banners, flyers and all my printing needs as well as being a great friend.
www.handy-office.co.uk

J Van Marle – For the awesome cover picture 'Purple Castle' – Conwy Castle.
www.jvanmarle.com

Lindsay Burgess – For hosting our Host for Hope event, Chester and ongoing support as a friend.
www.thepaintrepublic.com

Llandudno Bay Hotel – For letting us host our event and for going purple.
www.llandudnobayhotel.com

Llandudno Pier – For letting us light it purple.
www.llandudnopier.com

Lynn Quigley – North West Co-ordinator from Pancreatic Cancer UK.

Maggie and Roy Jenkins – Walking and supporting Martin on Wheelbarrow challenge.

Mama Life Magazine – A big shout out to Mel and Tash from Mama Life Magazine for featuring a full page pre-launch write-up in the Christmas 2018 issue.
www.mamalifemagazine.co.uk

Mark Phillips – For organising a wheelbarrow for our race and for donating some gifts on behalf Tesco in Llandudno Junction. Also for giving me permission to have a book signing at the store to show support and respect to Martin and for Pancreatic Cancer UK.

Mikyle, Charlie and Jennah – My children have been my reason for staying strong and positive.

Quay Hotel, Deganwy, North Wales – For hosting the Book Launch.
www.quayhotel.co.uk

Rebecca Lee – My special long-term friend, she supported the events, knitted Mr Hedgehog, sang at our events and has been there for me too.

Sarah Watkins – For arranging the Rydal Penrhos Choir Charity event and to all those for supporting it.

Svitlana Bulava from Green Pages UK for hosting our events in Chester and supporting the Purple Lights of Hope.
www.mygreenpages.co.uk

Tansy Rogerson – For helping organise Host for Hope events at LLandudno Bay Hotel.

Tom Spence – A Classical Cross-over Singer, who supported us at our Chester Gala Awards event with Green Pages UK.
www.tom-spence.com

Tony and his beloved wife Jennifer (RIP) **Wetherill** friends and supporters of the Wheelbarrow challenge.

The Crowne Plaza Hotel and Esther Events for supporting the Gala Awards Awareness event in Chester.

Veena Jain aka 'Storm V' – For agreeing to perform a Bollywood and Bhangra dance performance for the book launch.

Welsh Mountain Zoo – For lighting the entrance purple and also being part of the Wheelbarrow Story.
www.welshmountainzoo.org

My mum for keeping me strong with her prayers, especially on Fridays.

All the wheelbarrow participants for taking part, raising funds and keeping the campaign positively purple and fun.

A big THANK YOU to my Ucan2 Global Partners Dave Ives, Grahame J Brown, Jason Regan, Peter Webb and our Ucan2 family for their love, support, donations and the respect they have given me.

To all our friends near and far for their love, support with beautiful messages to donations that poured in worldwide.

ABOUT THE AUTHOR

Ghazala Jabeen is a mum of three and lives on the beautiful coast of North Wales, UK.

She is the Founder of her award-winning business Bollywood Burnout with her unique Bollywood and Bhangra style fitness programme. She is known to many as the 'The Bollywood Queen'.

She has been recognised as an international female speaker attending many public speaking duties at many events, radio stations and also runs a 'Lady Leaders Global' group to help inspire other women to lead the way in business. She has written for publications like Mama Life Magazine, a foreword for her friend Philippa Gitten's book and many other online and offline training programmes as well as being featured in many newspaper articles and appearances on TV.

She was awarded an Ambassador for Direct Sales and Network Marketing Industry award from Business for Home at the European Congress in Amsterdam and featured on the Hall of Fame 2018 with BFH. She is a Presenter and a Motivational Speaker with her own vibrant unique style.

She is also a President with World Global Network together with her business Partners at Ucan2 Global. She is a Sales and Media Marketing Trainer. She coaches people from all walks of life from personal development, online business growth to personal fitness. The other title she goes by is 'The Marketing Machine'.

Her closest work has been community projects and charity work especially with her own chosen charity Pancreatic Cancer UK after losing her husband to this dreadful cancer. She has raised thousands of pounds for this charity as well as other charities.

Ghazala is a very strong, driven and a positive lady that takes any task with a hands-on approach and goes the extra mile to see her commitment through.

Her own favourite quote is 'Together let's make a mark as we make a difference'. This is her first self-published book and is sure to make a mark.

www.ghazalajabeen.co.uk
www.justgiving.com/gaz-jabeen

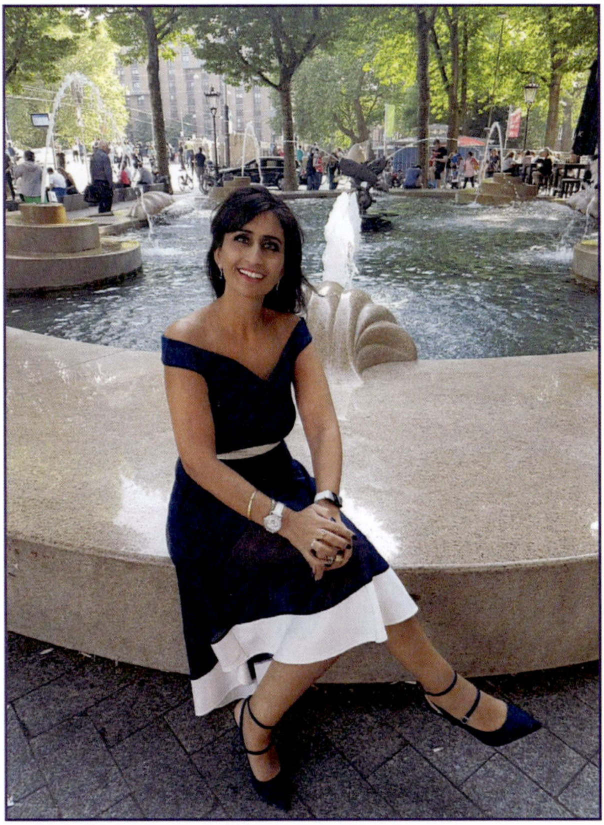

PANCREATIC
CANCER
AWARENESS

MR. H.M.S